Bone Marrow Diagnosis:
An illustrated guide

Bone Marrow Diagnosis:
An illustrated guide

David Brown
Department of Histopathology
Whittington Hospital
London
UK

Kevin Gatter
Nuffield Department of Clinical Laboratory Sciences
John Radcliffe Hospital
Oxford
UK

Yasodha Natkunam
Department of Pathology
Stanford University School of Medicine
Stanford, California
USA

Roger Warnke
Department of Pathology
Stanford University School of Medicine
Stanford, California
USA

Second edition

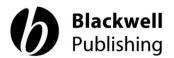

© 2006 David Brown, Kevin Gatter, Yasodha Natkunam and Roger Warnke
Published by Blackwell Publishing Ltd
© 1997 Blackwell Science Ltd
Blackwell Publishing, Inc., 350 Main Street, Malden, Massachusetts 02148-5020, USA
Blackwell Publishing Ltd, 9600 Garsington Road, Oxford OX4 2DQ, UK
Blackwell Publishing Asia Pty Ltd, 550 Swanston Street, Carlton, Victoria 3053, Australia

The right of the Author to be identified as the Author of this Work has been asserted in accordance with the Copyright, Designs and Patents Act 1988.

First published 1997
Second edition 2006

2   2008

Library of Congress Cataloging-in-Publication Data

Bone marrow diagnosis : an illustrated guide / David Brown ... [et al.].
  – 2nd ed.
    p. ; cm.
  Rev. ed. of: An illustrated guide to bone marrow diagnosis / Kevin Gatter, David Brown. c1997.
  Includes bibliographical references and index.
  ISBN: 978-1-4051-3561-0
  1. Bone marrow—Diseases—Diagnosis. I. Brown, David, M.D
  II. Gatter, Kevin. Illustrated guide to bone marrow diagnosis.
    [DNLM: 1. Bone Marrow Diseases—diagnosis—Atlases. 2. Bone
  Marrow Diseases—pathology—Atlases. WH 17 B712 2006]
  616.4'1075—dc22

                                                                    2006005809

A catalogue record for this title is available from the British Library

Set in 10/12pt Minion by the Medical Informatics Unit, NDCLS, University of Oxford
Printed and bound in India by Replika Press Pvt. Ltd

Commissioning Editor: Maria Khan
Editorial Assistant: Jennifer Seward
Development Editor: Elisabeth Dodds
Production Controller: Kate Charman

For further information on Blackwell Publishing, visit our website:
http://www.blackwellpublishing.com

The publisher's policy is to use permanent paper from mills that operate a sustainable forestry policy, and which has been manufactured from pulp processed using acid-free and elementary chlorine-free practices. Furthermore, the publisher ensures that the text paper and cover board used have met acceptable environmental accreditation standards.

Contents

Preface to the second edition

Eight years on from our first edition it is surely time for an update. The biggest expansion is in the author list bringing onboard the expertise of the Pathology Department at Stanford. The aims of the book remain the same as before: a simply written and well-illustrated text for the busy diagnostician. All the cases come from our own services and none have been worked up specifically for this book. In fact virtually all of the images are straight off the routine immunostainer. We continue to use Giemsa staining even though the rest of the world seems not to bother and in spite of the increased repertoire of antibodies which some think make histology stains, even the beloved H&E, redundant. We don't think so and unless you have unlimited resources, how do you know which antibodies to order unless you look at a well stained section first?

Once again there are so many people without whom a book like this could not be written that a full list would resemble the phone book. However, we'd like to mention Francesco Pezzella, Chris Hatton, Andy Peniket, Jim Wainscoat, Robin Roberts-Gant, Linda Summerville, Helen Turley, Letitia Campo, Kieron White, Paul Allen, Peter Isaacson and Norman Parker.

D. Brown, K.C. Gatter, Y. Natkunam and R. Warnke

Preface to the first edition

It has been said that the best way to travel is hopefully. Perhaps this is also the best way to write a textbook though I doubt that many authors begin in that way. We set out to write this book on bone marrow pathology because we thought we could write the sort of text that we would want to use ourselves. An inordinate amount of time later and suitably humbled we doubt that we ever want to see this manuscript again. Nevertheless it still approximates to the goal we were seeking. A short text oriented at diagnosis and comprehensively accompanied by usable illustrations. Our aim was to enable a busy pathologist to find on one open page the essential description and illustration of most common bone marrow diseases seen in trephines. We hope we have been successful but welcome comments and criticisms from readers. Who knows we might even produce another edition!

Acknowledgments

It is almost impossible to know where to begin when paying tributes and compliments to one's tutors and colleagues. Many indeed may not want the dubious honour of such recognition. It is impossible to learn anything about bone marrow without the help and tolerance of hematologists so we thank all the many colleagues we have worked with in Oxford over the years. We are both indebted to many histopathologists who tried to teach us the critical examination of tissue slides but all of whom recoiled in horror at looking at trephines. So we are substantially self taught and can only blame ourselves. Three individuals who have stimulated us in different ways often unknowingly need a special mention. They are Michael Dunnill, David Mason and Peter Isaacson. Our thanks to them and to all the others.

The text and image manipulation has all been performed in house in the Department of Cellular Science. This is still a relatively new technology for us and we would not have made any progress without our excellent medical informatics unit run by Kingsley Micklem. We owe a great debt of gratitude to Felicity Williams and Ellie Parker who performed all of the technical work on this project.

K.C. Gatter and D.C. Brown

Chapter 1 Introduction

During the late 1950s, McFarland and Dameshek introduced an acceptable means of obtaining bone marrow core biopsies.[1] This advance made it possible for the histopathologist to diagnose a wide range of hematopathologic disorders including the leukemias, lymphoproliferative and myeloproliferative disease, myelodysplasia, metastases and reactive disorders.

Most biopsies are taken from the posterior superior iliac spine. Ideally, in an adult, the core of tissue should be at least 1 cm in length. An aspirate is usually taken from the same site before the biopsy is removed (but from a different needle track or the biopsy may be a hemorrhagic mess). The hematologist will usually make about 10 smear preparations from the marrow particles that have been aspirated and either discard or send the remainder for histology. We find it useful to have both of these types of specimen because there are occasions when only an aspirate is available, in which case it is then important to have built up experience examining aspirate preparations for which trephines have been available for comparison.

The trephine biopsy has a number of advantages over the aspirate specimen. The most important is to enable examination of the topographic distribution of the cellular constituents of the marrow, their relationships to the bony trabeculae and an assessment of marrow cellularity. Furthermore, in diseases that produce fibrosis (e.g. Hodgkin lymphoma or myeloproliferative disorders) an aspirate often fails to produce an adequate diagnostic sample ("a dry tap").

Close liaison with hematologists is important because it makes the reporting of trephine biopsies easier and ensures that misdiagnoses are kept to a minimum.

There has been debate involving the embedding medium for bone marrow biopsies. There are essentially two schools of thought: those who believe that the biopsies should be embedded in plastic and those who believe paraffin embedding with decalcification to be superior. The reason for this divergence is related to the nature of the biopsy itself which consists of both hard tissue (i.e. bone) and soft tissue (i.e. marrow and fat). In order to cut intact sections one can either make the biopsy material uniformly soft (by decalcification) or uniformly hard (by resin embedding).

Unfortunately, decalcification inevitably produces some tissue distortion and plastic embedding limits the range of immunohistochemical studies. The debate over which is superior continues with vociferous advocates on both sides.[2–6] The advantages and disadvantages of each approach are shown in Table 1.1.

Table 1.1 Comparison of the relative advantages and disadvantages of paraffin and plastic embedding of bone marrow trephine biopsies.

	Paraffin embedding	Resin/plastic embedding
Advantages	1 Widespread antigen preservation allows immunohistochemical studies 2 Pathologists are familiar with sections cut from paraffin embedded material	1 Superb cytologic detail available from the very thin sections obtained by this technique
Disadvantages	1 Loss of some histochemical reactivity within the granules of the granulocyte and mast cell series, e.g. Leder stain. This loss is directly proportional to the strength of the acid used in decalcification 2 Some inevitable tissue distortion is produced by decalcification	1 Loss of some immunoreactivity 2 A separate technique is required solely for bone marrow biopsies 3 Pathologists are unfamiliar with resin embedded sections and their associated artefacts, e.g. the basophilic hue indicative of erythroid histogenesis is lost in resin embedded sections

We believe that, with a little extra care, it is possible to provide sections from paraffin embedded trephines that meet the practical requirements of the diagnostic hematologist.[7]

Just as there has been division amongst some pathologists regarding the best embedding medium so too has there been debate over which is the most appropriate general stain. This inevitably involves an element of personal preference. The well-established place of the hematoxylin and eosin (H&E) stain in general diagnostic pathology has assured it of much support amongst pathologists as the primary stain in bone marrow histology. We believe that a good Giemsa stain provides more information than its H&E counterpart, e.g. in identifying cell lineage, the detection of fibrosis and the estimation of iron stores. A good Giemsa stain requires fastidious technical preparation (see Chapter 12). The results are worth the initial perseverance on both the part of the technical staff and the pathologist who has to become familiarized with it. When indicated we include a reticulin stain in our bone marrow set.

Reasons for performing bone marrow biopsies

The majority of bone marrow biopsies are performed for the following reasons.[8]

1 Dry tap. The most common diagnoses are:
   - fibrosis (Hodgkin lymphoma, metastatic cancer, primary myelofibrosis);
   - hairy cell leukemia;
   - extreme hypercellularity ("packed marrow") such as may be seen in cases of leukemia and lymphoma.
2 Assessment of cellularity:
   - extent of infiltration by leukemia, lymphoma and myeloma;
   - amount of residual marrow;
   - assessment of marrow post chemotherapy and after engraftment;
   - investigation of cytopenias.
3 Identification of focal disease:
   - metastatic cancer, lymphomas, granulomas.
4 Lymphoma staging.
5 Assessment of HIV and its opportunistic infections.

How to examine a trephine section

It is important to have an organized approach to the examination of bone marrow sections in order not to miss diagnostic features. One possible scheme is based on an assessment of cellularity, topography, morphology and accessory structures as illustrated in Tables 1.2–1.5 with a selection of some common pathologic conditions.

Table 1.2 Assessment of cellularity with some common pathologic conditions as examples.

Cellularity	Conditions
Hypocellular	Aplastic anemia
	Hairy cell leukemia
	Acute myeloid leukemia
Normocellular	Be aware of subtle infiltrates such as myeloma
Hypercellular	
Homogeneous	Non-Hodgkin lymphoma
	Acute leukemias
	Reactive
Heterogeneous	Myeloproliferative syndromes
	Myelodysplasias
	Metastatic cancer
	Small cell tumors of childhood

Table 1.3 Topography (distribution) of cellular elements

Are all cell types present?
Are any particular cells present in abnormal numbers?
   e.g. increased granulocytes in chronic granulocytic leukemia
   prominent mast cells in Waldenström macroglobulinemia

Normal cellular distribution
Granulocytes
   Paratrabecular, peri-arterial
Erythroid
   Intertrabecular
Megakaryocytes
   Intertrabecular and peri-sinusoidal

Common abnormal patterns
Myelodysplasia/myeloproliferation
   Paratrabecular erythroid and megakaryocytic colonies
   Megakaryocytic clustering
Non-Hodgkin lymphoma
   Follicular lymphoma has a paratrabecular pattern
   CLL is usually diffuse or nodular

Table 1.4 Assessment of cell morphology.

Atypia
Abnormal megakaryocytes in myeloproliferation and myelodysplasia

Maturation abnormalities
Maturation arrest, e.g. drug induced
Asynchronous maturation in myelodysplasia
Abnormal maturation, e.g. megaloblastic anemia
Imbalance of maturation, e.g. left/right shifted

Table 1.5 Assessment of accessory structures.

Vessels
Vasculitis
Amyloid deposition

Sinusoids
Distended in myeloproliferative disorders

Bone
Osteoporosis
Osteomalacia
Paget disease

Stroma
Iron deposition
Amyloid
Gelatinous transformation
Granulomas
Fibrosis
Metastatic carcinoma
Gaucher disease

Organisms
Mycobacteria (TB)
Atypical mycobacteria
Leishmania
Histoplasma
Cryptococci

An historical aside

Later on in this book there is some discussion about the change of name given to Hodgkin's disease by the recent World Health Organization (WHO) classification committee. The authors of this text thought readers might be interested in Thomas Hodgkin, who was a true medical character of his time and involved in many more activities than pure pathology.[9] He described his eponymous disease in 1832 but by the 1840s had more or less abandoned medicine for philanthropy. He ended up in Jaffa, Israel in 1866 on a humanitarian mission with Sir Moses Montefiore where he died of infectious disease, probably cholera. His grave (Fig. 1.1—erected by Sir Moses) is tucked away behind the British school and is well worth a visit.

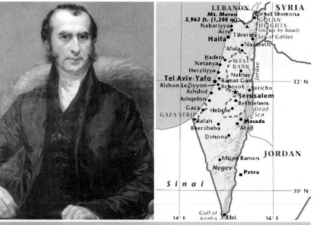
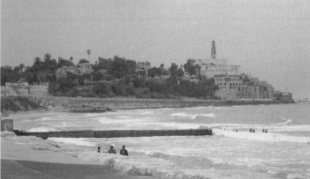
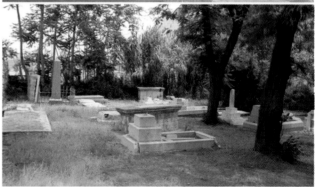
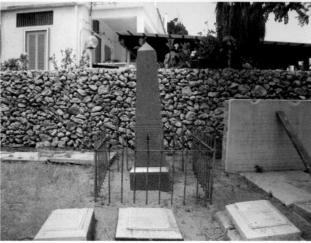

Fig. 1.1 Montage showing Thomas Hodgkin about the time of his description of his lymphoma. He is buried in Jaffa, Israel in a tiny cemetery behind the British school.

References

1 McFarland W, Dameshek W. Biopsy of bone marrow with the Vim-Silverman needle. *JAMA* 1958; **166**: 1464–6.

2 Hand NM. Misunderstandings about methyl methacrylate. *J Clin Pathol* 1993; **46**: 285.

3 Jack AS, Roberts BE, Scott CS. Processing of trephine biopsy specimens. *J Clin Pathol* 1993; **46**: 285–6.

4 Schmid C, Isaacson PG. Bone marrow trephine biopsy in lympho-proliferative disease. *J Clin Pathol* 1992; **45**: 475–50.

5 Schmid C, Isaacson PG. In reply to correspondence. *J Clin Pathol* 1993; **46**: 285–6.

6 Krenacs T, Krenacs L, Bagdi E. Diagnostic immunocytochemistry in Araldite-embedded bone marrow biopsies. *Cell Pathol* 1996; **1**: 83–8.

7 Gatter KC, Heryet A, Brown DC, Mason DY. Is it necessary to embed bone marrow biopsies in plastic for haematological diagnosis? *Histopathology* 1987; **11**: 1–7.

8 De Wolf-Peeters C. Bone marrow trephine interpretation; diagnostic utility and pitfalls. Invited review. *Histopathology* 1991; **18**: 489–93.

9 Rosenfeld L. Thomas Hodgkin: *Morbid Anatomist & Social Activist.* New York: Madison Books, 1992.

Chapter 2 The normal bone marrow

The bone marrow is not a random mixture of different blood-forming cells but is a highly organized and specialized tissue. The identification of individual cells is less precise in trephines than smear preparations because of the greater cytologic detail present in the latter. Consequently, a proportion of the marrow cell population will only be identifiable by the "company it keeps" or by special staining procedures, notably immunocytochemistry (e.g. stem cells cannot be identified morphologically).[1] Confidence in examining a trephine biopsy is derived from a familiarity with the normal marrow appearances and an understanding of how these alter throughout life.

Site of hematopoiesis

In the normal adult, hematopoiesis is largely restricted to the axial skeleton (i.e. skull, sternum, vertebrae, ribs, pelvis and the proximal regions of the long bones). The marrow in these sites is described as red because of the presence of erythroid elements and in the non-hematopoietic sites as yellow because of the large amount of fat present. Site and cellularity vary with age (Table 2.1 and Fig. 2.1).

Table 2.1 Bone marrow cellularity.

Age	Site	Cellularity (hemopoietic cells/fat)
Neonate	All bones, liver, spleen	100/0
Child	Most bones	70/30
Adult	Axial skeleton	50/50
Old age	Axial skeleton	30/70

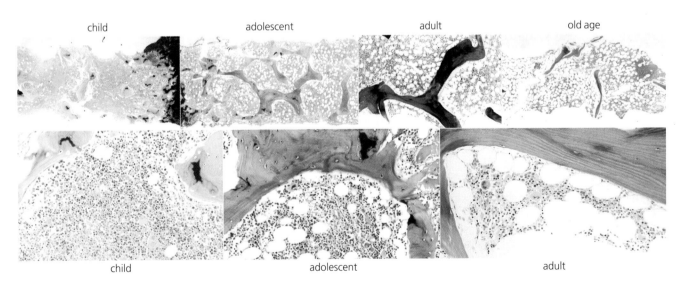

child   adolescent   adult   old age

child   adolescent   adult

Fig 2.1 Examples of bone marrow cellularity at different ages

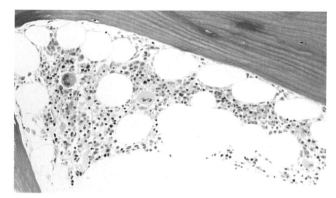

Fig 2.2 Lamellar bone showing parallel lines of ossification. Giemsa.

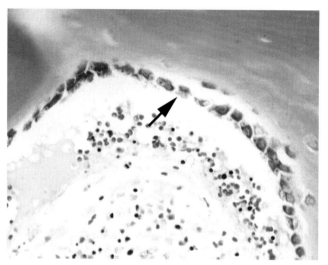

Fig 2.3 Osteoblasts (arrow) along the endosteal surface. Giemsa.

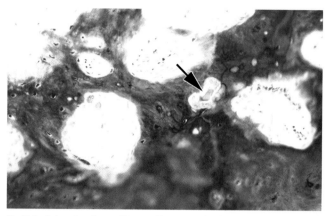

Fig 2.4 Osteoclast (arrow) housed in a Howship lacuna. Giemsa.

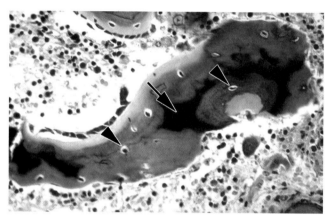

Fig 2.5 Cartilage (arrow) undergoing ossification. Osteocytes (arrowheads) are present within the lacunae. Giemsa

Components of the normal bone marrow trephine

- Bone
- Stroma: vessels, reticulin, fibroblasts, fat, iron
- Hematopoietic tissue: granulocytic, erythroid, megakaryocytic
- Other cells: lymphoid, plasma cells, mast cells

Bone

The trabeculae consist of lamellar bone (Fig. 2.2). Osteoblasts are present along the endosteal surface (Fig. 2.3). These may superficially resemble plasma cells because of the eccentrically placed nucleus and the presence of a cytoplasmic hof (paranuclear area of lighter staining cytoplasm). Osteoblasts lack the characteristic "clock face" nuclear chromatin pattern of plasma cells and the hof of the osteoblast does not abut directly onto the nucleus, but is separated by a narrow rim of darker staining cytoplasm.

Multinucleated osteoclasts are also present at the endosteal surface and within Howship lacunae (Fig. 2.4). These cells normally possess 4–6 nuclei but their number can increase in certain conditions (e.g. Paget disease). In young patients where remodeling of the bone is occurring at a high rate, osteoblasts and osteoclasts can be easily identified. In prepubertal patients, where fusion of the epiphyses has not yet occurred, cartilage undergoing ossification is usually present (Fig. 2.5).

Osteocytes are easily identified within their lacunae (Fig. 2.5). They have densely stained irregular nuclei and because of retraction artefact do not completely fill the lacunae. In necrotic or non-viable bone the osteocytes die and disappear (Fig. 2.6). In elderly patients with osteoporosis the trabeculae are thinned (i.e. generally less than the diameter of a fat cell) (Fig 2.7).

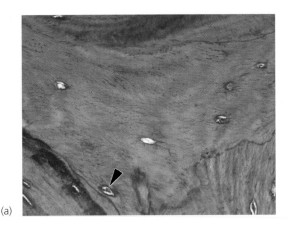

(a)

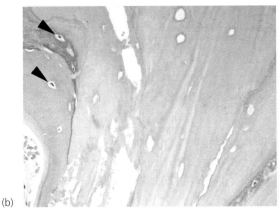

(b)

Fig 2.6 (a) and (b) Necrotic bone. Note the absence of osteocytes in the lacunae. There is a small focus of viable bone where osteocytes are present (arrowheads).

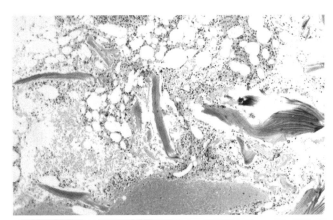

Fig 2.7 Typical example of thin trabeculae in the osteoporotic bone of an elderly patient. Such trephines are often rather shattered in appearance as they tend to crumple up on biopsy due to the weakness of the bone.

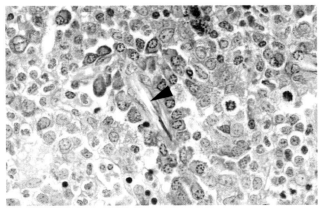

Fig 2.8 Small capillary (arrowhead) surrounded by a thin layer of mature plasma cells. Giemsa.

Stroma

Vessels

Thin-walled venous sinusoids are present throughout the marrow. In the normal marrow they are inconspicuous because they are usually collapsed. This is in contrast to those seen in the myeloproliferative syndromes where they may be dilated and prominent. They act as the efferent pathway for the mature hematopoietic elements on their way into the general circulation. Mature megakaryocytes are often seen close to or abutting onto the thin walls of these sinusoids, into which they discharge their platelets (Fig. 2.23). Small arteries may also be seen and identified by their relatively thick muscle walls. Granulopoiesis may be seen in proximity to them. Capillaries are easily seen and may be surrounded by a single layer of mature plasma cells, particularly in reactive conditions (Fig. 2.8).

Reticulin and fibroblasts

The blood-forming areas of the normal adult marrow have little reticulin and no fibrosis (i.e. fibrosis is regarded as an increase in the number of single reticulin fibers or bundles of fibers to form collagen). The reticulin is produced by inconspicuous elongated fibroblasts and exists as a fine network throughout most of the marrow although it may be condensed and more prominent around arterial vessels. The Gomori silver stain for reticulin readily displays this fine reticulin network, which can be graded semi-quantitatively when abnormal (Fig. 2.9).

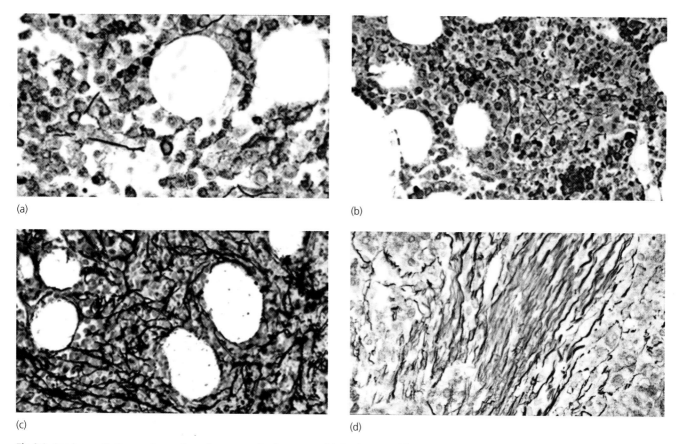

(a)

(b)

(c)

(d)

Fig 2.9 Semi-quantitative grading system of marrow reticulin content. (a) Grade 1. Focal fine reticulin. Normal. Gomori. (b) Grade 2. Diffuse fine reticulin. Normal. Gomori. (c) Grade 3. Diffuse fine reticulin, plus focal coarse reticulin. Abnormal. Gomori . (d) Grade 4. Diffuse coarse reticulin including collagen (i.e. fibrosis). Abnormal. Gomori.

Key points

- Increased fine and coarse reticulin is present around thick-walled blood vessels.
- Aspirated fragments of marrow tend to contain less reticulin than trephine biopsies. This is because those areas in a marrow with the least reticulin are the most easily aspirated.
- Crush artefact with smearing and elongation of cell nuclei produces a histologic picture that may mimic fibrosis (Fig. 2.10).
Silver staining is required for differentiation.

Fat

The amount of fat within red marrow increases with age, and consequently the amount of hemopoeitic tissue decreases (Fig. 2.11). In a section of trephine from a normal adult, the fat occupies approximately 50% of the marrow space. The subcortical region of the iliac crest has a greater percentage of fat than deeper regions and hence biopsies containing tissue from the subcortical region should not be misdiagnosed as hypocellular or aplastic. Similarly, there is considerable variation in cellularity throughout a trephine biopsy, a feature that emphasizes the need for an adequately sized biopsy (>1 cm) that will permit an accurate assessment of the marrow's cellularity. In the normal marrow the cellular elements are separated from the endosteal surface by a single layer of fat cells often referred to as the "first fat space" (Fig. 2.12). Fat atrophy may occur in hypothyroidism.

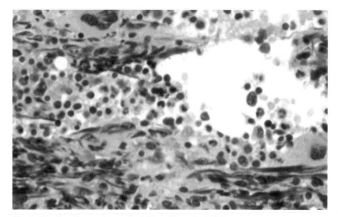

Fig 2.10 Crush artefact mimicking fibrosis. H&E.

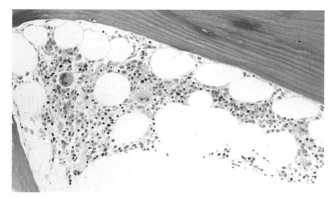

Fig 2.12 Single layer of fat cells separating marrow from the endosteal surface "first fat space." Giemsa.

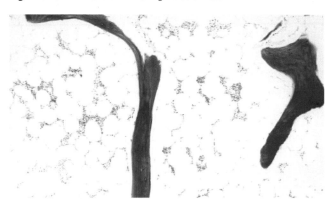

Fig 2.11 Marrow from elderly patient showing increased fat. Giemsa.

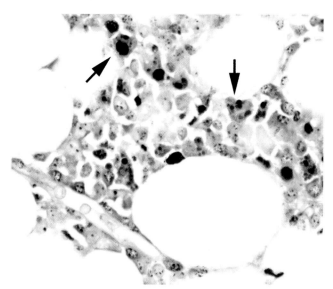

Fig 2.13 Post blood transfusion marrow showing how well Giemsa staining highlights iron in macrophages (arrows).

Iron

Perls' Prussian blue, which stains hemosiderin, will allow a semi-quantitative assessment of the amount of iron in marrow macrophages. Decalcification causes some loss of iron so that, when indicated, iron stains should be performed on both the aspirate and the trephine biopsy (some authorities only stain the aspirate for this reason). The Giemsa stain also identifies hemosiderin, producing an olive green coloration of the iron granules (Fig. 2.13).

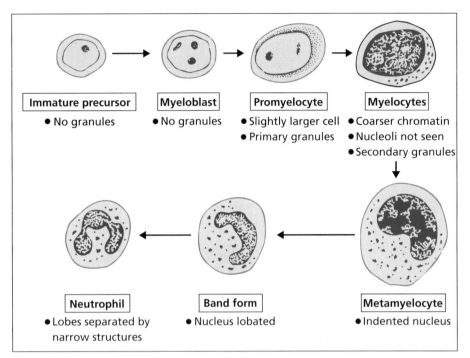

Fig 2.14 Schematic illustration of granulocytic cell differentiation.

Hematopoietic tissue

The granulocytic series (Fig. 2.14)

Immature forms of the granulocytic series are arranged along the endosteal surface of the trabeculae with maturation occurring towards the central intertrabecular region (Fig. 2.15).

A similar arrangement can also be seen around small arteries within the marrow (Fig. 2.16). Eosinophil precursors can be identified and distinguished from neutrophil precursors by their coarser granules which tend to be refractile and a darker red. Immunohistochemistry can be useful in identifying these cells (although not as yet in distinguishing the various types of myeloid cells).

The normal adult marrow has a granulocyte : erythroid ratio of approximately 2 : 1, as assessed by tissue section. In the first few weeks after birth, infants have a reversed ratio with up to 70% of the cells being of the erythroid series, mainly pro-erythroblasts and normoblasts.

The normal mature neutrophil has up to five nuclear lobes. In tissue sections fewer lobes are seen than in smear preparations because the latter allow whole intact cells to be visualized. In tissue sections, if more than three lobes can be identified the neutrophil should be considered hypersegmented. The number of these forms is increased in megaloblastic anemia.

In marrows with increased numbers of neutrophils, such as in systemic infections or as a reaction to some malignancies (e.g. Hodgkin lymphoma), the granulocyte series is described as right-shifted. Alternatively, an increase in immature forms (e.g. in an early regenerating marrow or severe infection) is described as left-shifted. A left-shifted granulocytic series is often seen in neonates where promyelocytes and myeloblasts are more obvious than in adult marrow.

A paradox may occur where a patient has a raised white cell count in the peripheral blood but the marrow appears normal. This may be due to administration of steroids which cause demargination of polymorphs from vessel walls into the blood stream.

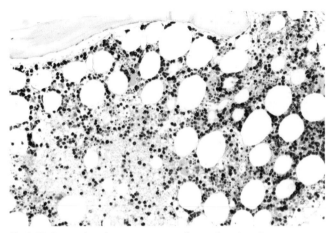

Fig 2.15 Paratrabecular arrangement of granulocytic series immunostained for myeloperoxidase.

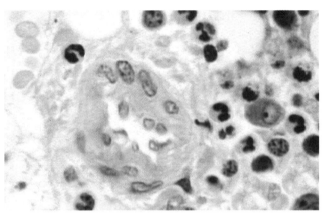

(a)

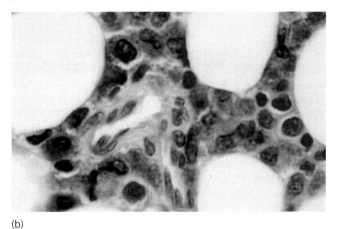

(b)

Fig 2.16 Arteriole with adjacent granulopoiesis.
(a) Giemsa. (b) Immunoperoxidase for elastase.

Table 2.2 Causes of erythroid hyperplasia.

Peripheral red cell loss or destruction
      e.g. hemorrhage
      e.g. hemolytic anemia
Ineffective erythropoiesis
      e.g. red cell membrane defects
      e.g. abnormal hemoglobin
      e.g. nutritional deficiency
Administration of erythropoietin

The erythroid series (Fig. 2.17)

Erythroid elements are organized into small groups present within the central regions of the marrow and extending up to the first fat space. Within these erythroid islands, all of the elements of this series can be identified, from the early pronormoblast (pro-erythroblast) through to the normoblast (late erythroblast).

Associated with many erythroid islands is a macrophage, usually located centrally and often containing free stainable iron (Fig. 2.18).

The Giemsa stain imparts a characteristic blueness (Fig. 2.19) to the blast forms of the erythroid series, a feature that is of use in distinguishing them from other immature cell types. This can be helpful in situations such as a marrow regenerating after chemotherapy when the possibility of residual leukemia is being considered. Paraffin embedding, but not plastic embedding, produces an artefactual halo around normoblasts, which is useful in distinguishing them from small lymphocytes (Fig. 2.20).

The normal marrow of a neonate may contain multiple groups of erythroid cells, which should not be misinterpreted histologically as metastatic disease (Fig. 2.21).

Erythroid hyperplasia is not uncommon (Table 2.2). Confusion may arise because, in this setting, the erythroid series may show some megaloblastic change. Furthermore, the large numbers of normoblasts present may create a monotonous histologic picture superficially similar to chronic lymphocytic leukemia (CLL). Immunohistochemistry can be particularly valuable in identifying cells of the erythroid series.

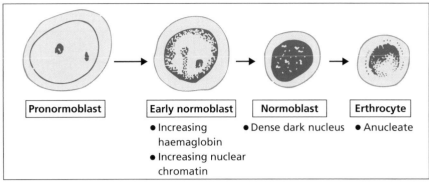

Fig 2.17 Schematic illustration of erythroid differentiation.

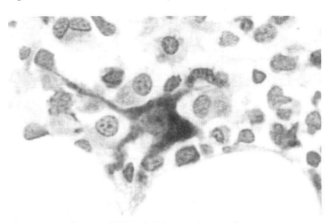

Fig 2.18 Small erythroid island with central macrophage immunostained for CD68. Immunoperoxidase.

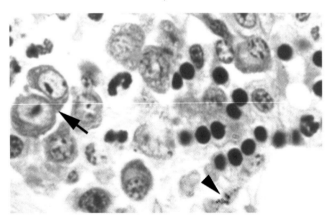

Fig 2.19 Erythroid colony showing distinct blueness of erythroblasts (arrow). Note also haemosiderin stains green (arrowhead). Giemsa.

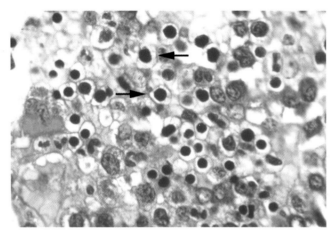

Fig 2.20 Normoblast (arrows) showing "halo" artefact. Giemsa.

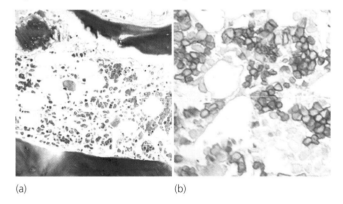

(a)   (b)

Fig 2.21 Neonatal marrow showing erythroid colonies which should not be confused with metastatic disease. (a) Giemsa. (b) Immunostaining for red cell glycophorin. APAAP (alkaline phosphatase:anti-alkaline phosphatase method).

Table 2.3 Megakaryocyte morphology in hematologic conditions.

Condition	Megakaryocyte morphology
Reactive	Emperipolesis
Idiopathic thrombocytopenic purpura	Increased numbers of small immature megakaryocytes
Myelodysplastic syndrome	Increased numbers of small (micro) megakaryocytes, diffusely arranged
Chronic myeloid leukemia	Increased numbers of small (micro) megakaryocytes, diffuse, small clusters
Essential thrombocythemia	Increased numbers of giant megakaryocytes, often in clusters
Polycythemia vera	Increased numbers of pleomorphic megakaryocytes, all sizes, clustered
Primary myelofibrosis	Increased numbers of pleomorphic megakaryocytes, all sizes, clustered

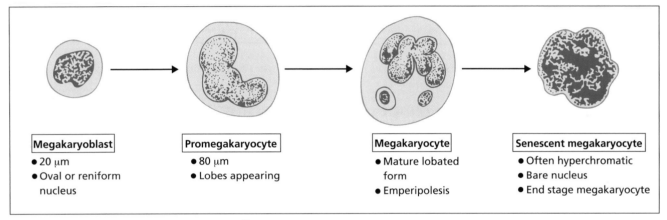

Megakaryoblast
- 20 μm
- Oval or reniform nucleus

Promegakaryocyte
- 80 μm
- Lobes appearing

Megakaryocyte
- Mature lobated form
- Emperipolesis

Senescent megakaryocyte
- Often hyperchromatic
- Bare nucleus
- End stage megakaryocyte

Fig 2.22 Schematic illustration of megakaryocytic differentiation.

The megakaryocytic series (Fig. 2.22)

Mature megakaryocytes and their precursors are found uniformly distributed throughout the central region of the marrow, particularly in association with thin-walled venous sinuses (Fig. 2.23).

Mature megakaryocytes do not usually occur in groups or lie in contact with each other. The presence of more than a few megakaryocytes close to bone trabeculae is abnormal. The mature forms are easily identified on tissue sections because they are the largest cells within the normal marrow. Less mature forms (e.g. megakaryoblasts) are less easily identified using conventional stains but are readily recognized immunohistochemically.

It should be remembered that in a histologic section one is seeing only a small part of a megakaryocyte and in order to obtain a reliable impression of megakaryocyte morphology many megakaryocytes should be examined. Emperipolesis (the safe passage of intact cells through the cytoplasm of another cell) is occasionally seen to occur in megakaryocytes. Although its significance is not known it is seen more frequently in reactive conditions and appears to be a non-specific feature (Fig. 2.24). Occasionally, megakaryocytes may be seen in mitosis (Fig. 2.25).

The term "pleomorphism" is used to describe megakaryocytes in a number of diseases, particularly the myeloproliferative disorders. Because normal megakaryocytes exhibit polyploidy there is an inevitable degree of nuclear pleomorphism in these cells. None the less, for diagnostic purposes, some megakaryocytes can be described as pleomorphic, in a pathologic sense, when variations in cell size, shape, nuclear morphology and topographic distribution exceed that seen in a normal marrow. Table 2.3 gives a summary of these changes.

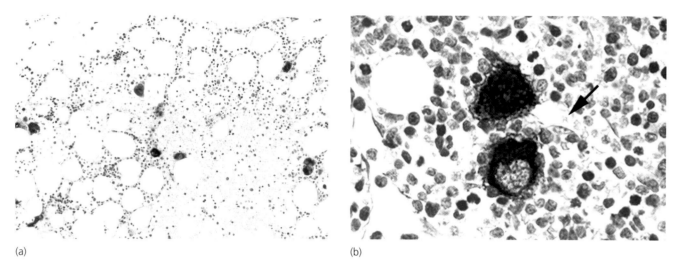

(a)   (b)

Fig 2.23 Distribution of megakaryocytes stained for CD61 in normal marrow: (a) low power view immunoperoxidase and (b) higher power view showing two megakaryocytes lying in close proximity to a venous sinusoid (arrow). APAAP.

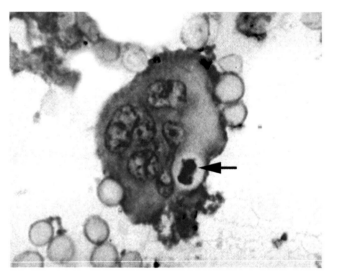

Fig 2.24 Megakaryocyte showing emperipolesis. A neutrophil (arrow) is present within the megakaryocyte. Giemsa.

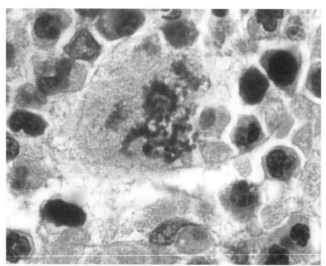

Fig 2.25 Megakaryocyte showing mitosis. H&E.

Table 2.4 A comparison of the features that may help discriminate between benign lymphoid aggregates in bone marrow and neoplastic involvement.

Benign	Neoplastic
Rounded aggregates	May be irregular
Well-circumscribed regular small lymphocytes	Cellular atypia may be present
Elderly population	Wide age range
<3 mm in diameter	May be >3 mm diameter
Rarely paratrabecular	May be paratrabecular
Germinal centers (5% of cases)	Germinal centers rare
May contain plasma cells and eosinophils	Usually just lymphoid cells
Polyclonal light chain expression	Monoclonal light chain pattern
1–3 aggregates per trephine	>3 aggregates per trephine

Other cells

A number of other cell types, which are not directly related to the hematopoietic tissues, can be identified on tissue sections. These include lymphocytes, plasma cells, mast cells and macrophages.

Lymphocytes

Normal adult marrow contains an inconspicuous population of both B and T lymphocytes throughout the marrow. On immunohistologic examination these can seem surprisingly numerous but are usually small cells distributed evenly and separately (Fig. 2.26). They may occur as small aggregates or nodules, typically solitary and located in the center of a marrow space (Fig. 2.27).

These lymphoid aggregates increase in number with age, being frequently seen in the elderly population. If there are more than three lymphoid aggregates per trephine, it suggests a neoplastic rather than a reactive process. Distinguishing between benign lymphoid aggregates and those that are neoplastic can be difficult and their significance remains unresolved (Table 2.4).[2–4]

Demonstration of monoclonality using light chain immunostaining or polymerase chain reaction (PCR) may be possible in a number of cases, although this does not mean that the patient will subsequently develop the clinical features of a lymphoma. This may be partly because many of these patients are elderly and will die of unrelated conditions. Interestingly, a recent molecular study of nodules in patients with a known lymphoma concluded: "Our study demonstrates the validity of PCR in distinguishing benign from malignant lymphoid infiltrates in bone marrow biopsies. However, because false negative PCR results do occur, morphology is still the gold standard in evaluating bone marrow involvement by non-Hodgkin lymphoma (NHL). For this reason PCR can only be considered as a useful complementary investigation."[5]

There is a more difficult problem with a paratrabecular lymphoid aggregate that is the characteristic site of early marrow involvement by follicular lymphoma (see chapter 8.6). Clonality testing is virtually impossible at present for these lesions and therefore objective evidence is lacking. There are those who have no doubt these are malignant but others, including the authors, waver. We have seen occasional cases over the the last 20 years that have not developed into lymphoma. So were they malignant? This of course leaves the final problem in the lap of our clinicians. What if we do demonstrate one or two minor clonal aggregates in the marrow? Should this affect their treatment or management?

Finally, in neonates the normal marrow contains a much increased number of lymphocytes, which may account for up to 50% of the marrow's cellularity.

Plasma cells

These are easily identified in normal adult marrow and form approximately 2% of the cell population in the marrow. They may occur singly, in small groups (2–3 cells) or, more commonly, in association with capillaries where they form a single layer around the vessel (Fig. 2.9). Immature and binucleate forms are uncommon. Plasma cells with intracytoplasmic accumulations of immunoglobulin (i.e. Russell bodies) may be found in both reactive and malignant plasma cells. Whether benign or malignant, plasma cells are well-demonstrated immunocytochemically either with antibody VS38 against p63 or with antibodies against CD138.

It is difficult, using morphologic criteria alone, to differentiate between a highly reactive plasmacytosis (Table 2.5) and a well-differentiated myeloma, as both conditions may display large numbers of plasma cells (Table 2.6).

Assessment of light chain expression (either immunohistochemically or by *in situ* hybridization) is easily performed on paraffin wax embedded specimens and is a valuable means of differentiating between these two conditions because myeloma displays light chain restriction.

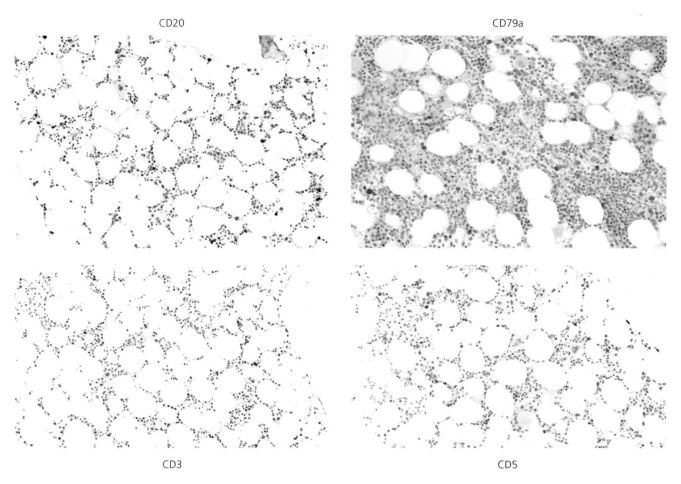

Fig 2.26 Distribution of B cells (immunostaining for CD20 and CD79a) and T cells (immunostaining for CD3 and CD5) in normal marrow. Immunoperoxidase.

Table 2.5 Causes of a reactive plasmacytosis.

HIV
Hepatitis
Systemic lupus erythematosus
Rheumatoid arthritis
Iron and folate deficiency
Alcohol abuse
Hodgkin lymphoma

HIV, human immunodeficiency virus.

Table 2.6 A comparison of the histologic features of reactive plasmacytosis and multiple myeloma.

Reactive plasmacytosis	Multiple myeloma
Majority are mature plasma cells	Variation in size and differentiation, intermediate forms common
Mainly mononuclear	Bi- and trinucleate forms common
Nucleoli uncommon	Nucleoli often present
No clusters	Clusters common
Single layer around capillaries	Several cells deep around capillaries

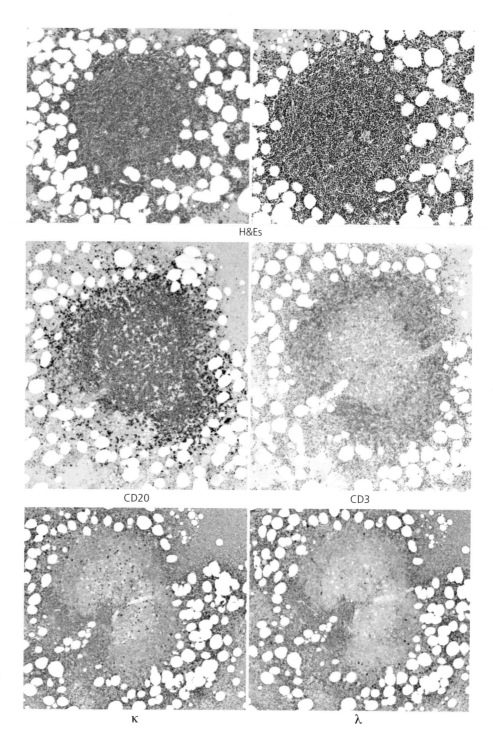

H&Es

CD20   CD3

κ   λ

Fig 2.27 Reactive lymphoid nodules in normal marrow (H&E) showing the distribution of B (CD20) and T (CD3) cells and the polyclonal nature of the B cells (κ and λ).

Mast cells

These are readily identified in tissue sections stained by Giemsa, where the metachromatic properties of the granules become apparent (Fig. 2.28). The cells have a round or oval nucleus and the cytoplasm contains many closely packed granules which have a dark blue appearance on Giemsa stained sections. They are distributed throughout the marrow with a tendency for a perivascular and paratrabecular distribution. They are increased in a number of lymphoproliferative disorders, particularly lymphoplasmacytic lymphoma (Waldenström macroglobulinemia) (Table 2.7). They are also usually easily detected by immunostaining for mast cell tryptase or CD117 (c-kit).

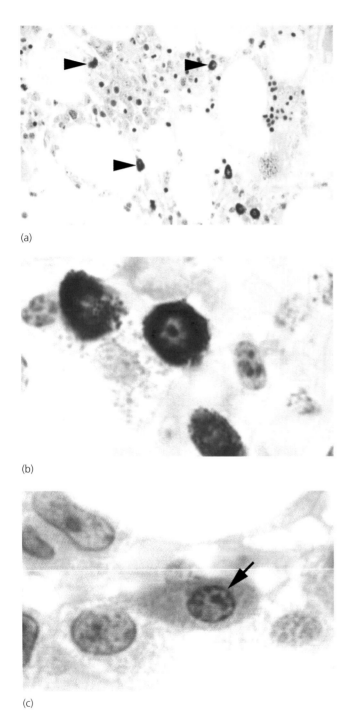

(a)

(b)

(c)

Fig 2.28 (a) A low power view of normal marrow showing scattered mast cells (arrowheads). (b) and (c) High power views showing (b) how Giemsa staining highlights mast cells which are often difficult to identify on (c) H&E (arrow).

Table 2.7 Causes of mast cell hyperplasia.

Lymphoproliferative disease, particularly Waldenström
   macroglobulinemia (lymphoplasmacytic lymphoma)
Alcohol excess
Radiation

Macrophages

Macrophages are present throughout the marrow, including the luminal surface of the sinusoids (Fig. 2.29). They are responsible for the phagocytosis and degradation of cellular debris produced by hematopoiesis and the removal of senescent cells. As such they contain iron, lipids and nuclear debris. Macrophages are clearly identified by immunostaining, with two of the best markers being CD68 and CD163.

Artefacts and unusual features

It is not uncommon to find that extraneous non-hematologic tissue has been introduced into the marrow during the biopsy procedure. This is usually epidermis although occasionally glandular appendages or muscle may be seen (Fig. 2.30). Sometimes a trephine might prove more difficult than usual to perform, resulting in traumatic hemorrhage into the marrow and disruption of its elements. Similar circumstances may also result in bone dust being introduced into the marrow producing a puzzling histologic appearance which can be misinterpreted as necrotic tissue unless the histopathologist is aware of this particular artefact (Fig. 2.31). Rarely, fully formed lymphoid tissue may occur in the marrow (Fig. 2.32).

In paraffin embedded tissues that have not been adequately decalcified or when the sections are cut particularly thin, bone trabeculae may be torn from the section during cutting. This leaves an empty space which resembles an ectatic sinus (Fig. 2.33). Unlike the sinus it lacks a continuous lining of endothelial cells and does not contain red blood cells. Crush artefact simulating fibrosis has been mentioned previously (see Fig. 2.10).

Fig 2.29 The distribution of macrophages throughout the normal marrow CD68 immunoperoxidase.

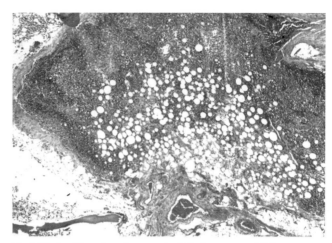

Fig 2.32 Small lymph node present within the marrow. H&E.

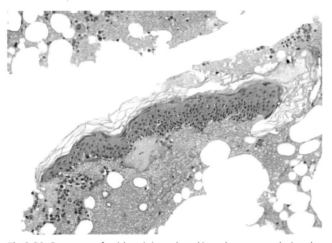

Fig 2.30 Fragment of epidermis introduced into the marrow during the biopsy procedures.

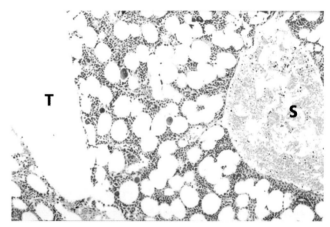

Fig 2.33 The space left by tearing out the bone trabecular (T) can look like a sinus (S) but lacks red cells and an endothelial lining. H&E.

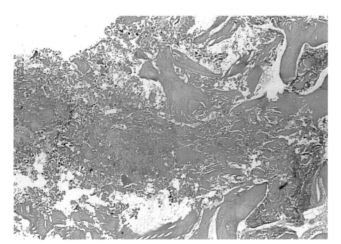

Fig 2.31 Bone dust filling the marrow cavity is an artefact of trephining. H&E.

References

1 Quesenberry PJ. The blueness of stem cells. *Exp Haematol* 1991; **19**: 725–8.

2 Rywlin AM, Ortega RS, Dominguez CJ. Lymphoid nodules of bone marrow: normal and abnormal. *Blood* 1974; **43**: 398–400.

3 Bartl R, Frisch B, Burkhardt R, *et al*. Lymphoproliferations in the bone marrow: identification and evolution, classification and staging. *J Clin Pathol* 1984; **37**: 233–54.

4 Faulkner-Jones BE, Howie AJ, Boughton BJ, Franklin IM. Lymphoid aggregates in bone marrow: study of eventual outcome. *J Clin Pathol* 1988; **41**: 768–75.

5 Maes B, Achten R, Demunter A, *et al*. Evaluation of B cell lymphoid infiltrates in bone marrow biopsies by morphology, immunohisto-chemistry, and molecular analysis. *J Clin Pathol* 2000; **53**: 835–40.

Chapter 3 Human immunodeficiency virus infection

Human immunodeficiency virus (HIV) infection may result in many changes to the bone marrow. These include reactive processes, secondary infections and the development of malignancies. They are a consequence of the virus's ability to impair the body's immune system. Some of the changes may be seen at a relatively early stage of HIV infection, before the onset of full-blown AIDS (acquired immune deficiency syndrome).

Clinical features

Within developed countries AIDS is predominantly associated with homosexuals and intravenous drug abusers and does not appear to have spread significantly into the heterosexual population as is the case in developing countries.

Consequently, most patients in the UK with HIV-related disease are young or middle-aged and male. They may present with a wide variety of complaints, the most common of which include weight loss, lymphadenopathy, diarrhea, oral thrush, cough, skin problems and general weakness. Aspiration of the marrow can be difficult.

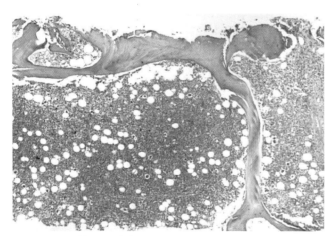

Fig. 3.1 Typical hypercellular marrow seen in uncomplicated HIV infection. H&E.

Reasons for performing bone marrow biopsies

Bone marrow changes are common in HIV-related disease. The cellularity is usually increased (Fig. 3.1) although approximately 20% of cases are hypocellular (Fig. 3.2).

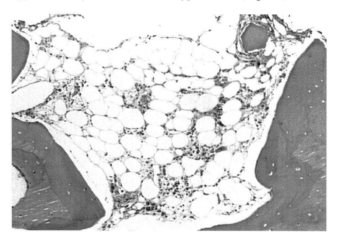

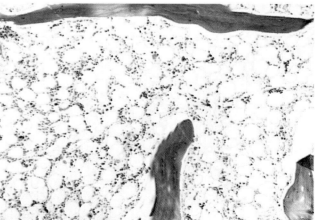

Fig. 3.2 Examples of hypocellularity seen in HIV infection. Top H&E, bottom Giemsa.

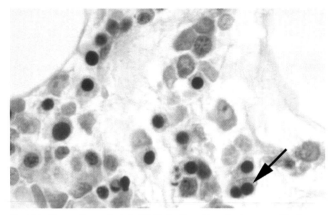

Fig. 3.3 Dyserythropoiesis in HIV infection. Binucleate normoblast (arrow). Giemsa.

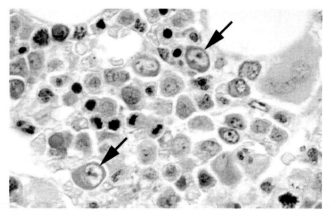

Fig. 3.4 Megaloblastic precursors (arrows) in HIV infection. Giemsa.

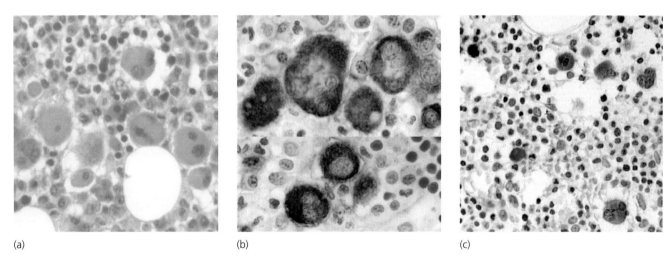

(a)   (b)   (c)

Fig. 3.5 Micromegakaryocytes in HIV infection. (a) Giemsa. (b) CD31. (c) CD61.

Reactive features

Up to three-quarters of HIV-infected marrows show dyshematopoiesis with myelodysplastic-like features affecting all three cell lines. Members of the granulocyte series may show nuclear abnormalities and decreased granularity. Eosinophilia is common (seen in 15% of cases). The erythroid series may show abnormalities of normoblast nuclei, especially binucleate forms and irregular nuclear outlines (Fig. 3.3) and occasionally megaloblastoid change is seen (Fig. 3.4).

The latter feature is said to be more common in patients taking zidovudine (AZT) where increased numbers of proerythroblasts with megaloblastic features are present. The megakaryocyte series shows increased numbers of micromegakaryocytes and mononuclear forms (Fig. 3.5).

Naked megakaryocyte nuclei are also seen and probably represent platelet-depleted (i.e. end stage) megakaryocytes (Fig. 3.6).

In addition to abnormalities involving hematopoietic tissue, considerable alterations to the stromal environment may also occur. Contributing to the hypercellularity of HIV-infected marrows are increased numbers of plasma cells, lymphocytes and macrophages (Fig. 3.7). Some of the latter may display erythrophagocytosis (Fig. 3.8).

The plasmacytosis can be particularly striking (Fig. 3.9) and easily mistaken for multiple myeloma. However, the plasma cells are polyclonal in nature, as demonstrated by light chain immunostaining. Aggregates of lymphocytes are not infrequent. Focal lesions consisting of loose, ill-defined aggregates of lymphoid cells, histiocytes and associated vascular proliferation may be seen and are known as lymphohistiocytic aggregates resembling those lesions seen in angioimmunoblastic T cell lymphoma (AITL) (Fig. 3.10). Conventional granulomas may be found in the absence of any obvious etiology.

Serous atrophy (gelatinous transformation) is frequently seen and when extensive the appearance is striking (Fig. 3.11). It is usually associated with more severe HIV-related disease that has involved rapid weight loss.

Giemsa

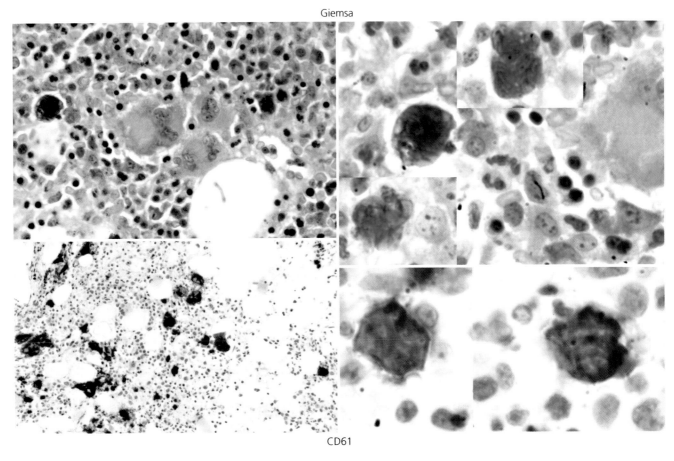

CD61

Fig. 3.6 Naked megakaryocyte nuclei. Giemsa and immunostains for CD61.

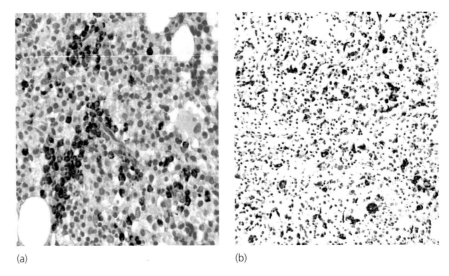

(a) (b)

Fig. 3.7 Increased numbers of plasma cells. (a) Antibody VS38 and macrophages. (b) Antibody against CD68 in HIV-infected marrow.

cytology   H&E

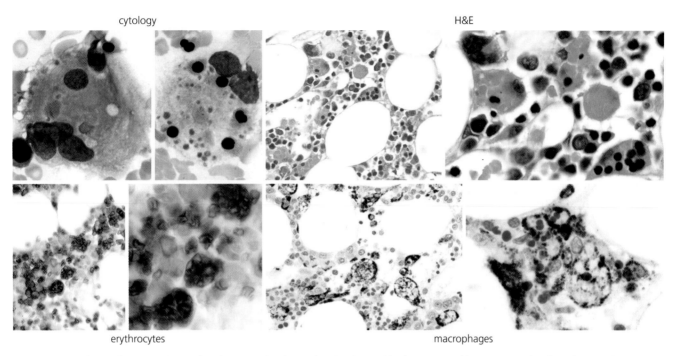

erythrocytes   macrophages

Fig. 3.8 Macrophages demonstrating erythrophagocytosis. The cytology is Giemsa, histology H&E and immunostains for glycophorin C showing the red cells and CD68 for macrophages.

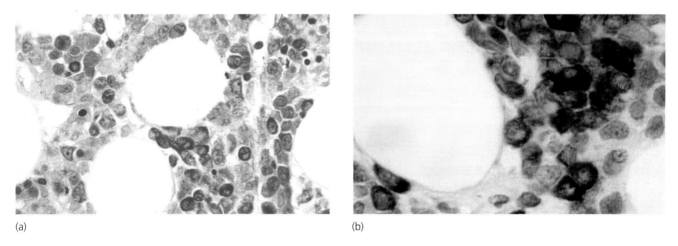

(a)   (b)

Fig. 3.9 Increased numbers of plasma cells. (a) Giemsa. (b) Antibody VS38.

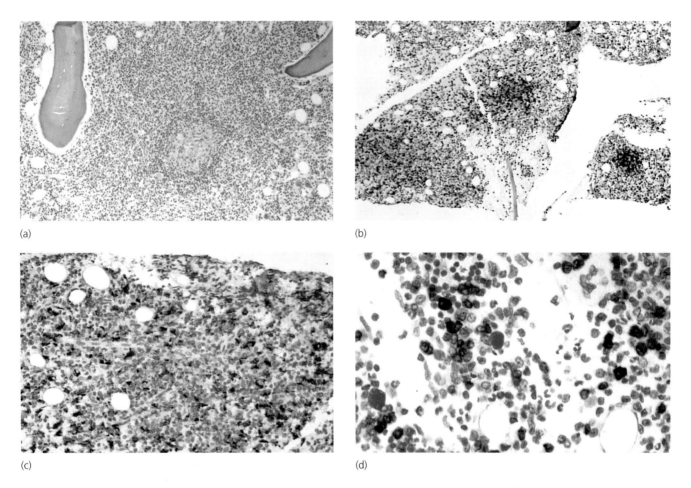

(a)

(b)

(c)

(d)

Fig. 3.10 Lymphohistiocytic aggregates in HIV. (a) H&E. (b) CD3 for T cells. (c) CD68 for macrophages. (d) CD79a for B lymphocytes and plasma cells.

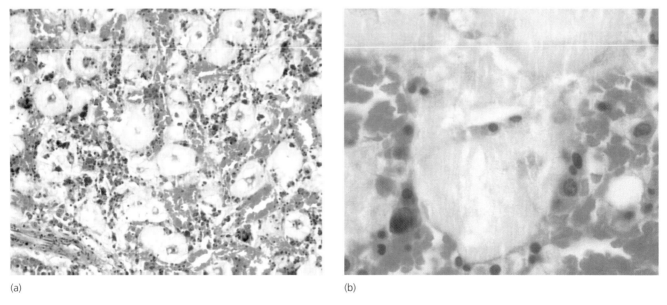

(a)

(b)

Fig. 3.11 Serous atrophy in HIV. (a) Low power. (b) High power. Both H&E.

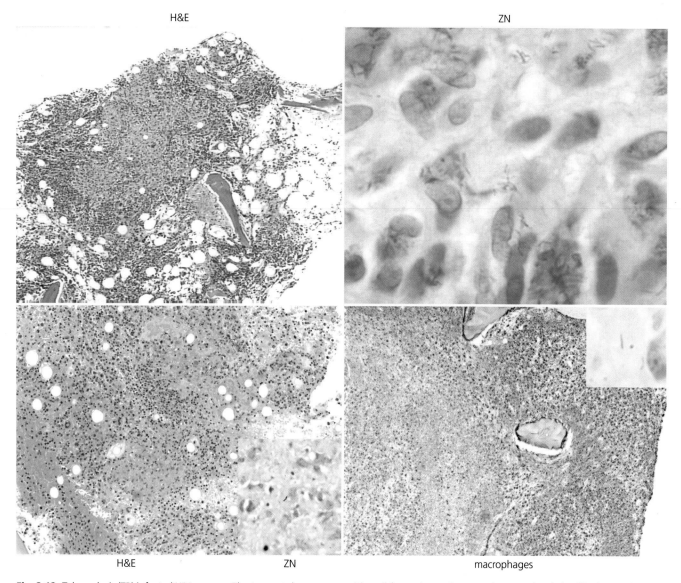

Fig. 3.12 Tuberculosis (TB) infected HIV marrow. The top row shows a case with well-formed granulomas and many tubercle bacilli whereas the lower row is a case with ill-formed granulomas but very few tubercle bacilli (shown in inserts). TB stained by Ziehl–Neelsen (ZN) and macrophages immunostained for CD68.

Secondary infections

These are common and patients often have multiple infections. The most commonly encountered are those involving acid-fast bacilli, usually tubercle bacillus (TB) or *Mycobacterium avium intracellulare* complex (MAIC). Granulomas are usually present in marrows infected by these organisms, although this is not always the case (Fig. 3.12). It is prudent to stain all known HIV marrow biopsies (and indeed all types of tissue biopsies from HIV-infected patients) with a Ziehl–Neelsen (ZN) stain, whether granulomas are present or not. The number of bacilli seen can vary considerably although large numbers are often present (Fig. 3.13).

The fungi *Cryptococcus* (Fig. 3.14) and *Histoplasma* (Fig. 3.15) and the protozoan *Leishmania* (Fig. 3.16) are usually found in reactive macrophages often associated with granuloma formation (Fig. 3.17). Cytomegalovirus (CMV) infection can be detected by characteristic nuclear inclusions, particularly within endothelial cells (Fig. 3.18). *Pneumocystis carinii* infection need not necessarily remain within the lungs and can become systemic, occasionally involving the bone marrow.[1]

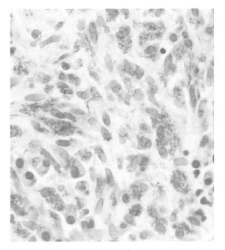

Fig. 3.13 Atypical tuberculosis in HIV marrow not associated with granulomas. ZN stain.

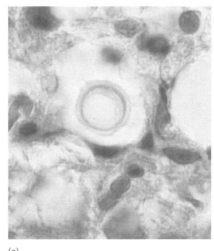

(a)

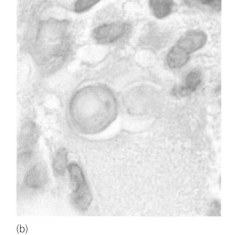

(b)

Fig. 3.14 HIV-associated cryptococcal infection. (a) H&E. (b) Mucicarmine.

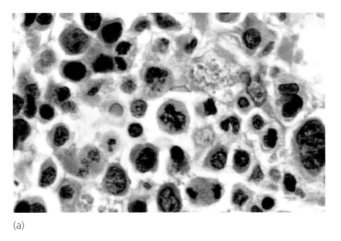

(a)

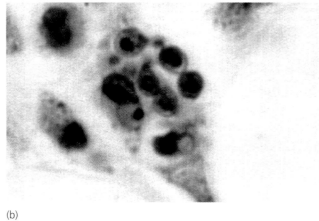

(b)

Fig. 3.15 HIV-associated histoplasmosis. (a) H&E. (b) Grocott.

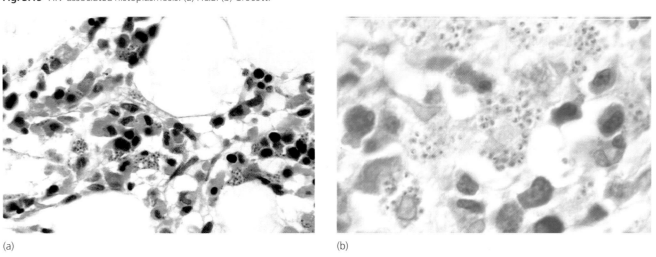

(a)

(b)

Fig. 3.16 *Leishmania donovani* bodies in macrophage cytoplasm. (a) H&E. (b) Giemsa.

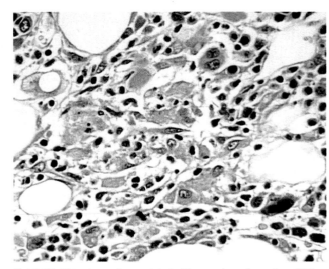

Fig. 3.17 Histoplasmosis associated with granuloma formation. H&E.

H&E   CMV

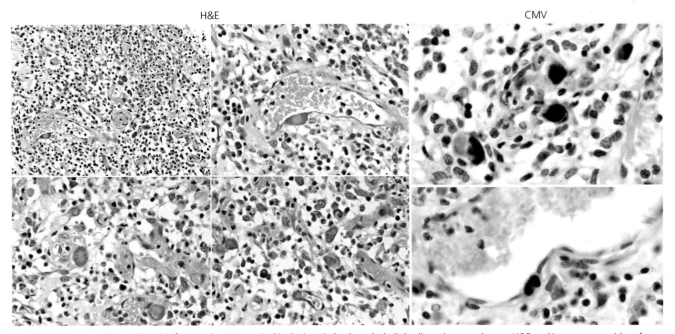

Fig. 3.18 Cytomegalovirus (CMV) infection showing typical inclusions in both endothelial cells and macrophages. H&E and immunoperoxidase for CMV.

Malignancies

Patients with HIV infection have an increased risk of developing a non-Hodgkin lymphoma. This is a high-grade malignancy often involving the marrow. It is usually of a B cell immunophenotype and has a large cell (centroblastic or immunoblastic) (Fig. 3.19), Burkitt (Fig. 3.20) or lymphoblastic morphology (Fig. 3.21). The subtyping of lymphomas in HIV infections is performed exactly as for those in non-HIV

infected individuals on both morphologic and immunophenotypic grounds as illustrated in the figures above (see Chapter 8 for more details).

Hodgkin lymphoma also appears to be increased in HIV-infected individuals (Fig. 3.22) and may have a more aggressive course than the conventional type.

Kaposi sarcoma can involve most organs including, rarely, the bone marrow (Table 3.1).

H&E Giemsa CD20

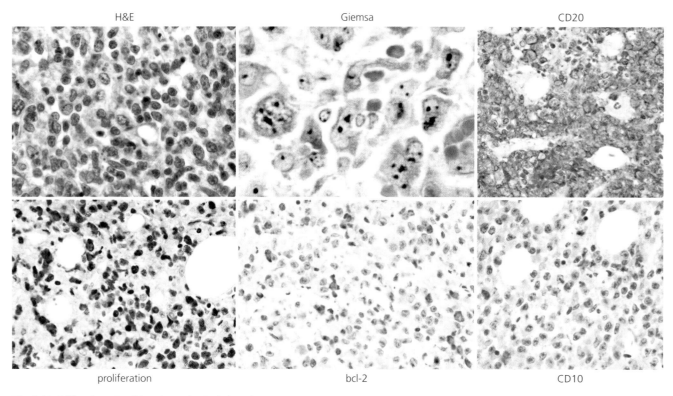

proliferation bcl-2 CD10

Fig. 3.19 Diffuse large B cell lymphoma in HIV-infected marrow.

H&E CD20

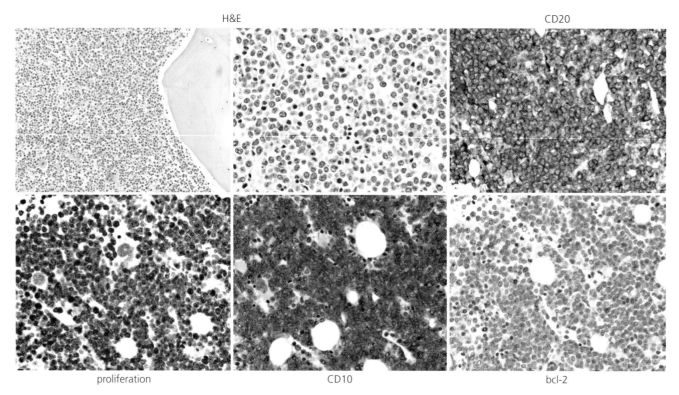

proliferation CD10 bcl-2

Fig. 3.20 Burkitt lymphoma in HIV-infected marrow.

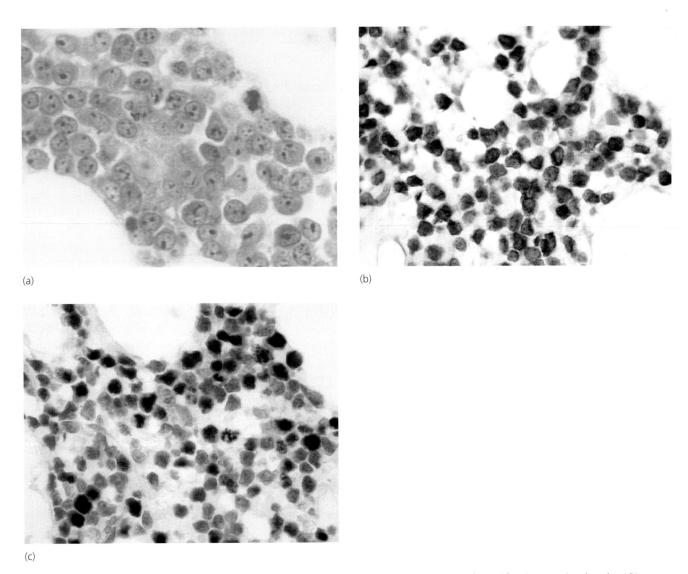

Fig. 3.21 B cell lymphoblastic lymphoma. (a) Giemsa. (b) B cell marker CD79a. (c) Immunoperoxidase for proliferation associated marker JC1.

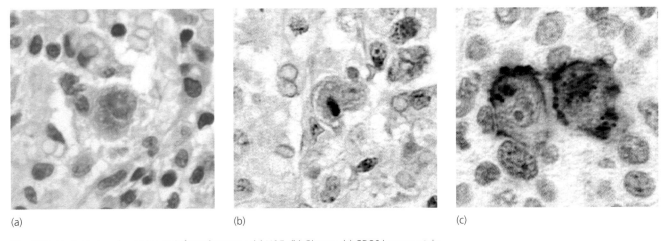

Fig. 3.22 Hodgkin lymphoma in HIV-infected marrow. (a) H&E. (b) Giemsa. (c) CD30 immunostain.

Table 3.1 Summary of features seen in HIV-positive bone marrow biopsies.

Myelodysplastic-like features	Stromal features
Seen in 75%	Increased plasma cells and macrophages
All three cell lines affected	Macrophages showing erythrophagocytosis
15% have eosinophilia	Serous atrophy
Megaloblastoid features	Lymphocytosis
Nuclear abnormalities in normoblasts	Lymphohistiocytic aggregates (AILD-like lesions)
Nuclear abnormalities and decreased	Vascular proliferation granularity in myeloid series
Micromegakaryocytes	
Mononuclear megakaryocytes	
Naked megakaryocyte nuclei	

Infections	Malignancies
Leishmaniasis	Kaposi sarcoma
Pneumocystis carinii	Non-Hodgkin lymphoma
Cryptococcus neoformans	Hodgkin lymphoma
Histoplasma capsulatum	
Mycobacterium avium intracellulare	
CMV	
TB	

AILD, Angioimmunoblastic T cell lymphoma; CMV, cytomegalovirus; TB, tuberculosis.

Diagnostic problems

1 Misdiagnosis as myelodysplastic syndrome (MDS) is unlikely because there are usually other features to suggest HIV infection. In addition, the clinical features including the patient's age would be unusual for a diagnosis of MDS.
2 A striking plasmacytosis may provide confusion with multiple myeloma. Immunohistochemistry will resolve this by demonstrating that the plasma cell population is polyclonal.
3 Megaloblastoid change seen in members of the erythroid series should not be misdiagnosed as leukemia or megaloblastic anemia, because the change is accompanied by other features of HIV infection.
4 Distinction between secondary infection by TB and by MAIC may be possible because MAIC tends to be periodic acid–Schiff (PAS) positive in addition to being ZN positive.

Key points

- Perform a ZN stain on all known HIV-infected marrow biopsies.
- HIV infection can cause a number of histologic changes, none of which are specific.
- Consider HIV infection in any marrow that shows ill-defined abnormalities that are not diagnostic of other conditions.

Reference

1 Telsak EE, Cote RJ, Gold JMW, *et al.* Extrapulmonary Pneumocystis carinii infections. *Rev Infect Dis* 1990; **12**: 380–6.

Chapter 4 Anemias and aplasias

Anemias

The majority of anemias are diagnosed and treated by a wide range of clinicians with only the more severe or complicated needing specialist hematological attention. Even then only a minority of these cases come to trephine biopsy. This reduces the pathologist's experience in these areas, which can lead to a misdiagnosis. This can be overcome to some extent by persuading the hematologist to submit the particles remaining after bone marrow aspiration for histopathology, even if no trephine is taken. The evaluation of marrow iron stores is an important consideration in the diagnosis of many anemias which is ideally performed on the bone marrow smear. It can be assessed on lightly decalcified sections processed promptly to paraffin and well stained by Giemsa, although one should be aware that some iron loss may occur during decalcification.

Iron deficiency anemia

Hematologists rarely examine the bone marrow in iron deficiency so that when trephines are taken they are often complicated by other clinical conditions. In uncomplicated iron deficiency anemia the marrow is usually slightly hypercellular due to increased erythropoiesis. Iron stores are reduced or absent (Fig. 4.1).

Anemia of chronic disease

Again trephines are not a first line of investigation in the anemias of chronic infections, inflammatory diseases or malignancy. The cellularity is normal or slightly reduced with iron detectable in macrophages (although many of these patients will have had blood transfusions) (Fig. 4.2).

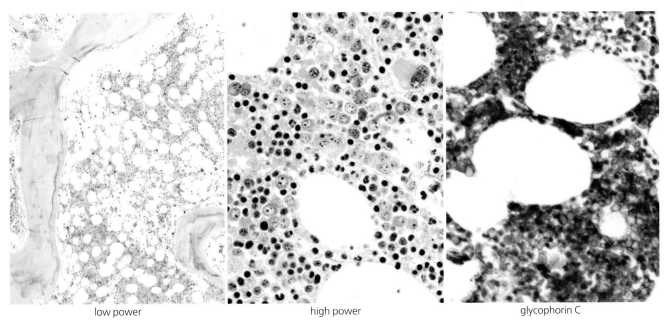

low power   high power   glycophorin C

Fig. 4.1 Iron deficiency anemia. Hypercellular marrow at low and high power showing increased erythropoiesis. Giemsa. Immunostained for glycophorin C to outline erythroid colonies.

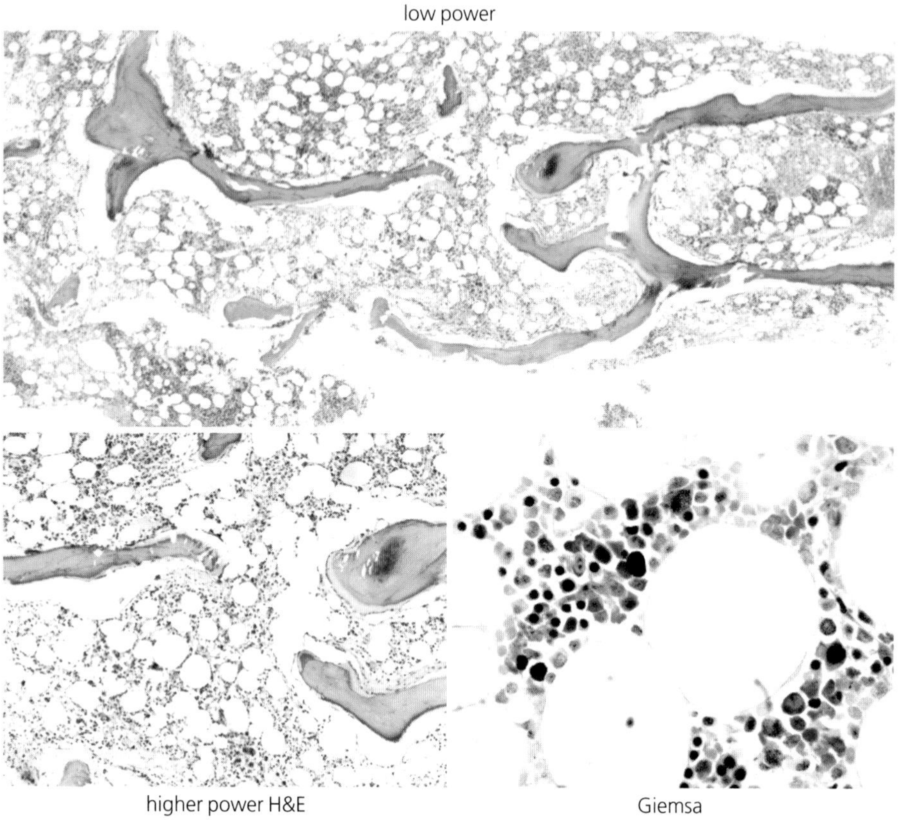

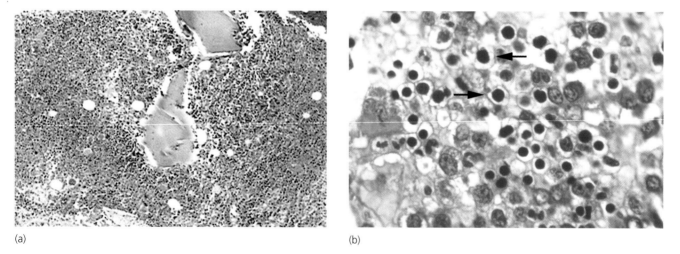

low power

higher power H&E

Giemsa

Fig. 4.2 Anemia of chronic disease. Normal cellularity for age shown at low and higher powers. H&E. Iron may be seen in macrophages staining green on Giemsa.

(a)

(b)

Fig. 4.3 Autoimmune hemolytic anemia. (a) Hypercellular marrow. (b) Erythroid hyperplasia. Giemsa.

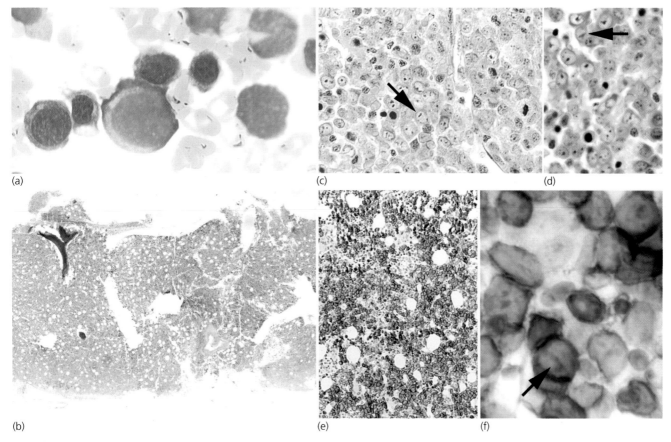

(a)

(b)

(c)

(d)

(e)

(f)

Fig. 4.4 Typical megaloblastic anemia. (a) Cytology. (b) Low power. (c,d) High power, (e,f) Immunostains for glycophorin C to highlight erythroid cells. Note the characteristic elongated "coin slot" nucleoli of the megaloblasts (arrows).

Hemolytic anemia

A trephine is usually taken to exclude an underlying malignancy such as chronic lymphocytic leukemia (CLL). Uncomplicated hemolytic marrows are hypercellular with marked erythroid hyperplasia but little else of note (Fig. 4.3).

Megaloblastic anemia

The marrow is usually hypercellular with loss of fat cells including the first fat space around the bone. The marrow is dominated by erythroid hyperplasia with significant left-shifting including the characteristic megaloblastic erythroid precursors(Fig. 4.4).

This and the cellularity may be so marked that it could be misdiagnosed as a malignancy such as leukemia, lymphoma or even carcinoma (Fig. 4.5). The diagnosis is easier to perform on an H&E because the deep blue cytoplasm of a good Giemsa often gives the game away. The other cell lines also demonstrate changes, most notably giant metamyelocytes in the granulocyte series. Occasionally, there may be such a significant increase in myeloid activity with associated blastic precursor cells that the picture can resemble acute myelocytic leukemia (AML) (Fig. 4.6).

These rare cases require careful clinical coordination.[1] Megakaryocytes are smaller, slightly increased in numbers and may have hyperlobated nuclei. These changes are typically caused by B_{12} or folate deficiency, although a number of drugs affecting DNA synthesis have also been implicated.

Other macrocytic anemias with many causes including drugs and alcohol can give rise to megaloblastic changes. The cellularity is usually normal or low without the dramatic picture of true megaloblastic anemia (Fig. 4.7).

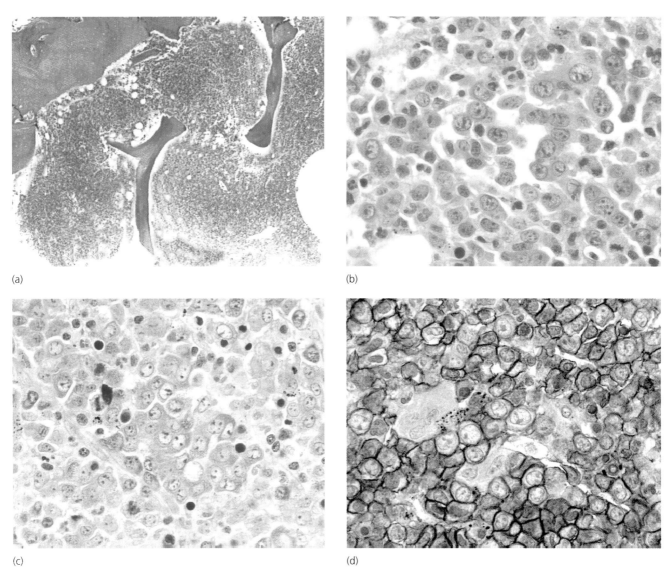

(a)

(b)

(c)

(d)

Fig. 4.5 Megaloblastic anemia with extreme hypercellularity with many blast cells simulating acute leukemia. (a) Low power. H&E. (b) High power. H&E. (c) High power. Giemsa. (d) Immunostain for red cell glycophorin. Peroxidase.

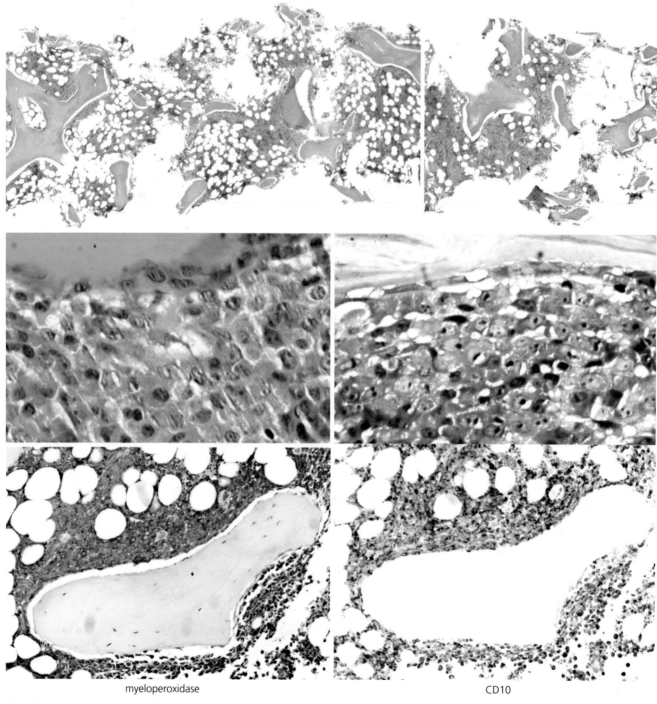

myeloperoxidase

CD10

Fig. 4.6 Megaloblastic anemia with extreme myeloblastic proliferation. Histology shown at low power with H&E and at higher powers with H&E and Giemsa, respectively. Immunostains for myeloperoxidase and CD10 highlight the paratrabecular aggregations of blasts. This case resolved with vitamin B_{12} administration.

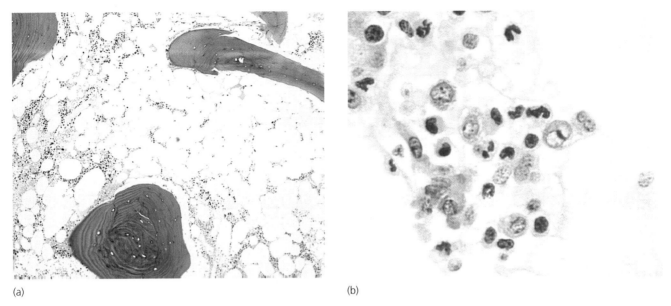

(a)   (b)

Fig. 4.7 Drug-induced macrocytosis. (a) Low power. (b) High power. Giemsa.

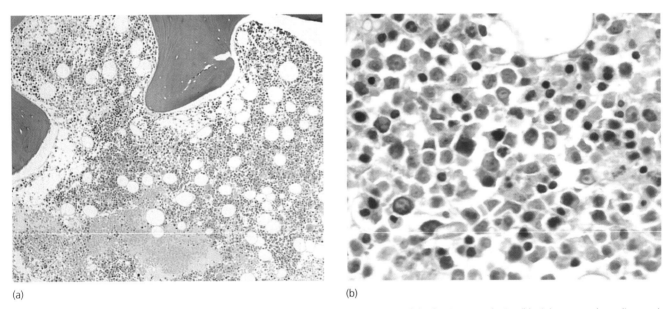

(a)   (b)

Fig. 4.8 Congenital dyserythropoietic anemia in a child's marrow. (a) Low power shown with both Giemsa and H&E. (b) High powers show disrupted erythroid colonies with marked pleomorphic features in all cell types, both by Giemsa and immunostaining.

Table 4.1 Drugs that may cause aplasia.

Type of drug	Example
Antibiotic	Chloramphenicol
Anti-inflammatory	Phenylbutazone
Antiepileptics	Phenytoin
Antimalarials	Mepacrine
Antidiabetic	Chlorpropamide

Congenital dyserythropoietic anemias

These are very rare inherited conditions which usually do not include a biopsy in their evaluation. The trephine is hypercellular, often with marked dyserythropoiesis and should always be considered in the differential diagnosis of dyserythropoiesis in children (Fig. 4.8).

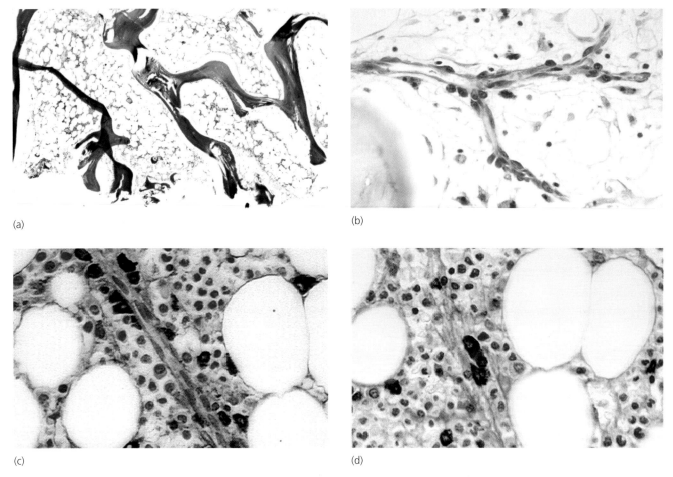

Fig. 4.9 Aplastic anemia. (a) Low power. Giemsa. (b) Vessel surrounded by reactive plasma cells showing polyclonal light chain production. (c) Kappa immunostain. (d) Lambda immunostain.

Aplasias

It is not easy to find a good definition for bone marrow aplasia. Possibly the best approach is to consider it a clinicopathologic correlation of profound cellular hypoplasia combined with pancytopenia. Fibrosis and malignant infiltration are usually excluded as causes.

Acquired aplastic anemia results from chemotherapy or wide field radiotherapy; the effect is dose related and inevitable. Many drugs can give rise to aplasia (Table 4.1) as will a variety of viral infections, especially hepatitis B and parvovirus. In a proportion of cases no obvious cause (often referred to as idiopathic cases) can be identified. Many of these are suspected to be hypocellular myelodysplastic syndromes and indeed there is evidence that approximately 10% of long-term survivors of aplastic anemia will go on to develop AML.[2]

Acquired aplastic anemias

The trephine features are similar regardless of the cause. The marrow is profoundly hypocellular although often focal areas of slightly increased cellularity may be seen. Inspection of these areas is often disappointing as they largely consist of inflammatory and stromal cells (Fig. 4.9).

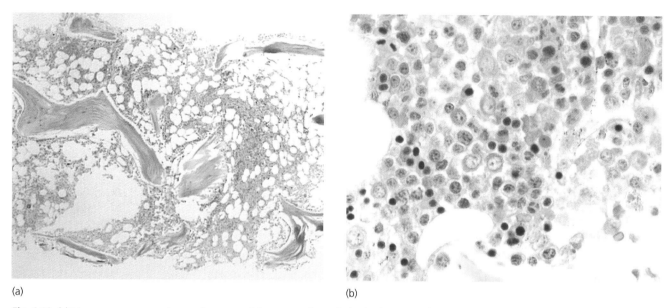

(a)   (b)

Fig. 4.10 (a) Marrow appearances 1 year after successful treatment for typical aplastic anemia. (b) High power view shows dysplastic changes (reduced granulocyte differentiation, dyserthropoiesis) which should not be interpreted as preleukemic. Giemsa.

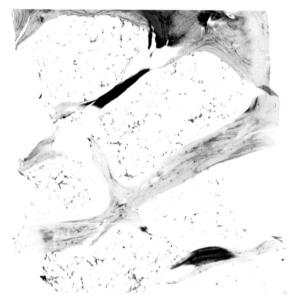

Fig. 4.11 Severely hypocellular marrow as seen in Fanconi anemia. Giemsa.

It is of course important to exclude hypocellular MDS/AML by ensuring that clusters of blast cells are not overlooked. With recovery, which may require steroid or growth factor treatment in idiosyncratic cases, there is frequently a period when the marrow appears profoundly dysplastic. One should be careful not to over-interpret this because given time the marrow will revert to a healthy state, especially in the post chemotherapy, viral or drug induced cases (Fig. 4.10).

Congenital aplastic anemias

There are a number of syndromes associated with congenital aplastic anemia either of all cell series (e.g. Fanconi syndrome) (Fig. 4.11) or of selective bone marrow series. Of the latter the Blackfan–Diamond syndrome shows pure red cell aplasia/hypoplasia (Fig. 4.12) and the Schwachman–Diamond (Fig. 4.13) is a form of granulocytic hypoplasia. All are rare and frequently managed without bone marrow histology. Fanconi anemia (and to a lesser extent Blackfan–Diamond) has a raised incidence of development of AML, which may be the first time the marrow is biopsied.

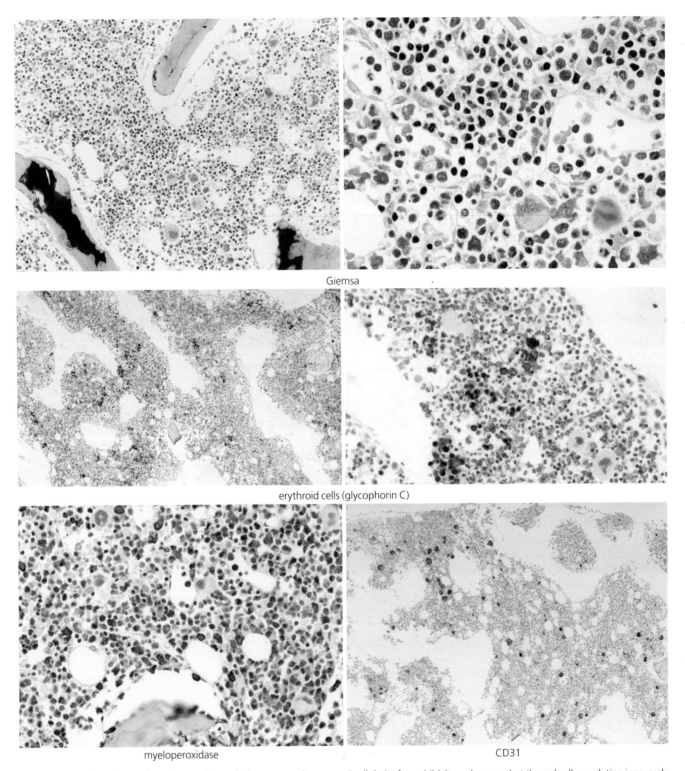

Giemsa

erythroid cells (glycophorin C)

myeloperoxidase

CD31

Fig. 4.12 Blackfan–Diamond syndrome. Although the marrow shows good cellularity for a child, it can be seen that the red cell population is severely restricted (Giemsa and glycophorin C immunostains) whereas granulocytes (myeloperoxidase) and megakaryocytes (CD31) are normal.

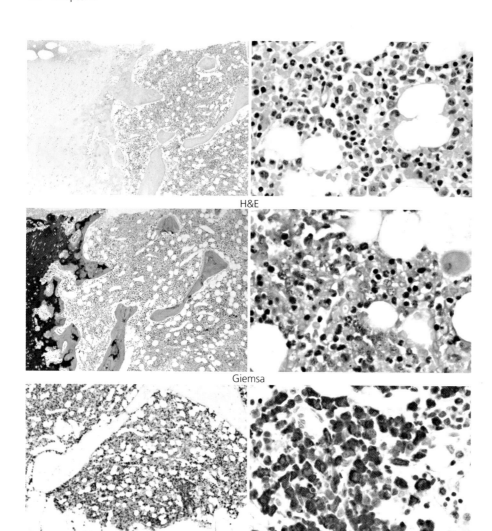

H&E

Giemsa

myeloperoxidase

Fig. 4.13 Schwachman–Diamond syndrome showing normal cellularity for age but with greatly reduced granulocytic maturation. Note that the myeloid population is relatively preserved and that it is the polymorph maturation that is heavily reduced.

References

1   Greer JP, Foerster J, Lukens JN, *et al.* (eds). Megaloblastic anemias: disorders of impaired DNA synthesis. In: *Wintrobe's Clinical Hematology*, 11th edition. Philadelphia: Lippincott Williams & Wilkins, 2003.

2   Gordon-Smith EC, Weatherall DJ, Ledingham JGG, *et al.* (eds). Aplastic anaemia and other causes of bone marrow failure. In: *Oxford Textbook of Medicine*, 3rd edition. Oxford: Oxford University Press, 1996.

Chapter 5 The myelodysplastic syndromes

A preleukemic state has been recognized for some time although different nomenclatures, e.g. "smouldering leukemia," "preleukemic syndrome" and "dysmyelopoietic syndrome," have given rise to some confusion. This situation has, to some extent, been clarified by the French–American–British (FAB) cooperative group who in 1982 proposed the term "myelodysplasia" and defined five subtypes.[1]

The more recent WHO classification of leukemias and lymphomas has more or less endorsed their subtyping with the following modifications. There is a new category of refractory cytopenia with multilineage dysplasia reflecting those cases with more dysplastic changes than are commonly seen in refractory anemia but where the blast count is less than 5%. Chronic myelomonocytic leukemia (CMML) is moved out of the myelodysplastic syndrome (MDS) category into a new category of "myelodysplastic/myeloproliferative disorders" reflecting the borderline nature of that condition. Refractory anemia with excess of blasts in transformation (RAEBt) is moved into the acute myeloid leukemias as AML with multilineage dysplasia which better reflects the clinical nature of this disorder. Finally, there are two new categories for unclassifiable cases and those cases previously classified with the refractory anemias but which possess an isolated chromosome 5 abnormality known as the 5q– syndrome.[2]

Although myelodysplasia is commonly thought of as preleukemic it should not be forgotten that most leukemias, particularly in children and young adults, develop *de novo*.

It should be emphasized that the FAB classification was designed to be used by hematologists not histopathologists and is not directly applicable to tissue sections where certain features are not apparent. For example, it is rarely possible to identify ringed sideroblasts in histologic sections of trephine biopsies.* This has not changed in the WHO classification where bone marrow histology is scarcely mentioned.

The inclusion of CMML as part of MDS is not universally accepted. Some authorities argue that it should be considered as an established leukemia and be placed with the myeloproliferative disorders.[3,4] As mentioned above, the WHO committee compromised and made a new borderline category for CMML.

Trephine biopsy plays an important part in the diagnosis of MDS and in monitoring its evolution, particularly when a dry tap is obtained (partly because the marrow is hypercellular and partly because of an increase in reticulin fibers). In addition, the histology provides information not available from a smear preparation, such as topographic abnormalities and changes to the marrow stroma. Indeed, it has become our view with experience that histopathology and histopathologists are not good at recognizing the different categories of MDS. Far and away our most important contribution is alerting clinicians to an impending transformation into AML when blastic activity is patchy and missed on the aspirate.

The FAB classification:

1 refractory anemia (RA);
2 refractory anemia with ringed sideroblasts (RARS);
3 refractory anemia with excess of blasts (RAEB);
4 chronic myelomonocytic leukemia (CMML);
5 refractory anemia with excess of blasts in transformation (RAEBt).

The WHO classification:

1 refractory anemia (RA);
2 refractory anemia with ringed sideroblasts (RARS);
3 refractory cytopenia with multilineage dysplasia (RCMD);
4 refractory anemia with excess of blasts (RAEB);
5 myelodysplastic syndrome, unclassifiable (MDS-U);
6 myelodysplastic syndrome with isolated del(5q) chromosome abnormality.

---

* These are erythroblasts with a ring of mitochondrial-associated free iron distributed around the nucleus and are probably related to the abnormal erythropoiesis seen in MDS.

Myelodysplasia

Clinical features

The typical picture is of an elderly patient (median 65 years) complaining of bleeding, recurrent infections or tiredness. These patients have an anemia that is unresponsive to iron supplements.

Hepato-splenomegaly and lymphadenopathy are not typical. The clinical course is variable; some patients progress to AML while others require little in the way of treatment. The majority of patients die from hemorrhage or sepsis.

The average survival for each group in the WHO classification is:

- RA   6 years
- RARS   6 years
- RCMD   3 years
- RAEB   14 months
- MDS-U   unknown

The 5q– syndrome has no significant effect on survival, having a very low transformation rate to acute leukemia.

Histopathology of the bone marrow

The appearances of MDS in tissue sections of the marrow consist mainly of loss of cellular differentiation and disruption of normal architecture. These changes can be considered analogous to those seen in premalignant conditions affecting other organs (e.g. cervical intraepithelial neoplasia, adenomatous polyps of the bowel and actinic keratoses). MDS is a stem cell disorder so that abnormalities may be apparent in any of the three blood-forming cell lines. It is a common misconception that marked abnormalities must be detected in each cell line in order to diagnose MDS on trephine sections. In fact the identifiable abnormalities may be restricted to only one series (e.g. the erythroid in sideroblastic anemia).

Cellularity

The marrow is hypercellular in the majority of cases (80%). In the remainder the marrow is normocellular or even hypocellular.

Abnormalities of marrow architecture

The most striking feature seen at low power is the disruption of the normal cellular distribution. The appearance is of all cell lines randomly mixed together rather than the normal orderly distribution of immature to mature cells from the bone towards the center. The marrow stroma is also altered. Edema, extravasation of red blood cells, sinus ectasia,

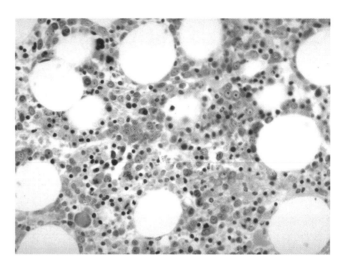

Fig. 5.1 Typical jumbled appearance of cell types in myelodysplasia. Giemsa.

increased reticulin formation, hemosiderin-laden macrophages, plasmacytosis and lymphoid aggregate formation all add to the anarchic appearance of MDS (Fig. 5.1). To appreciate these changes it is essential to have some knowledge of normal marrow histology.

Dysmegakaryopoiesis

The number of megakaryocytes is increased, which is best demonstrated immunohistochemically (Fig. 5.2). Their distribution is abnormal, with many having a paratrabecular location. A number of abnormalities in size, shape and nuclear lobe configuration may be present.

1 *Micromegakaryocytes.* These are normal in appearance except that the diameter of the cell is much reduced (Fig. 5.3).

2 *Monolobated megakaryocytes* (Fig. 5.4). These are not to be confused with megakaryoblasts which are normal precursors seen in a number of reactive conditions. Monolobated megakaryocytes are larger (>30 μm) than megakaryoblasts, have more cytoplasm (similar in amount to mature megakaryocytes) and a single-lobed nucleus without nucleoli. They are reported to be in increased numbers (>50%) in cases of MDS showing a deletion of all or part of chromosome 5q (the so-called 5q– syndrome[5]). This is of clinical relevance because patients with the 5q– syndrome have a lower incidence of leukemic transformation.

3 *Megakaryoblasts* (Fig. 5.5). These are increased in number and may be dysplastic. They are small, have a high nuclear : cytoplasmic ratio and the nuclei are hypolobated and may have nucleoli.

4 *Topographic abnormalities.* The main abnormalities are the paratrabecular distribution and clustering of two or more megakaryocytes with direct cellular contact ("kissing").

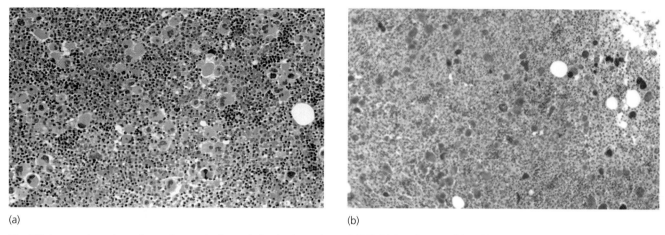

(a)   (b)

Fig. 5.2 Increased numbers of megakaryocytes in myelodysplastic syndrome (MDS). (a) Seen by H&E. (b) Highlighted by immunostaining for CD61.

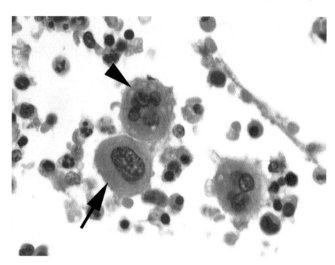

Fig. 5.3 Typical micromegakaryocyte (arrowhead) next to a monolobated form (arrow) in MDS. H&E.

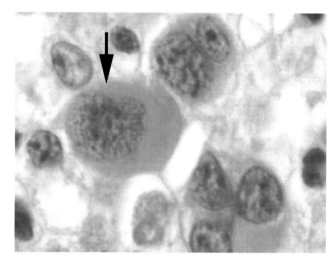

Fig. 5.5 Megakaryoblast (arrow) with two micromegakaryocytes. H&E.

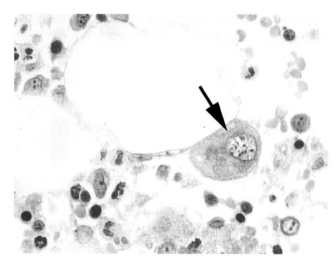

Fig. 5.4 Monolobated megakaryocyte (arrow) in MDS. Giemsa.

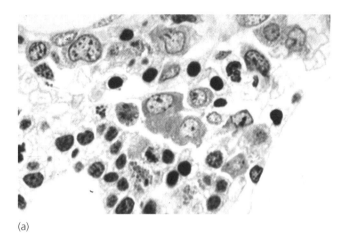

(a)

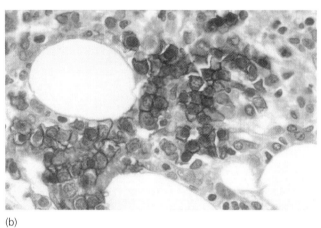

(b)

Fig. 5.6 Enlarged irregular erythroid colony in MDS highlighted by immunostaining for glycophorin C. (a) Giemsa. (b) Immunoperoxidase.

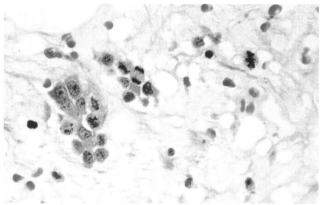

Fig. 5.7 Clusters of immature erythroid precursors in MDS. Giemsa.

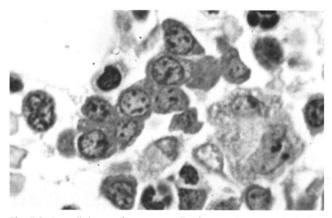

Fig. 5.8 A small cluster of precursor cells of uncertain origin which the authors believe represent abnormally located immature precursors (ALIPs). Giemsa.

Dyserythropoiesis

This is characterized by enlarged irregular erythroid colonies containing increased numbers of immature cells. These colonies lack the symmetry and central localization seen in normal marrows. These features may be highlighted by immunocytochemical staining for red cell antigens (Fig. 5.6). Frequently, the immature precursors are clustered together and are separated from the more differentiated erythroid cells by other marrow elements.

Cytologic abnormalities include binucleate or irregularly shaped normoblasts and megaloblastic precursors (Fig. 5.7).

Dysgranulopoiesis

A reduction in granulocytic maturation is usually evident although other abnormalities are less impressive than in the other cell series. Reduced cytoplasmic granulation and abnormalities of nuclear lobation are best appreciated in smear preparations.

Abnormally located immature precursors

Abnormally located immature precursors (ALIPs) are generally believed to represent primitive myeloid (i.e. granulocytic) precursors (Fig. 5.8). They are abnormal because of their location in the middle of the marrow and also because they occur in groups. They were reported to indicate a poorer prognosis because of a higher association with leukemic transformation.

This is a controversial area with strong advocates[6,7] and sceptics.[8–10] Part of the difficulty in resolving this dilemma lies in the subjective criteria for the recognition of ALIPs. Consequently there is no current consensus on their value in diagnosis.

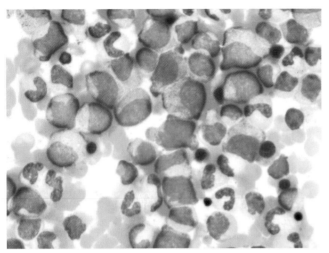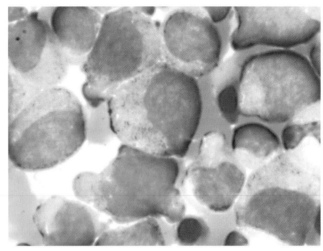

Fig. 5.9 The bone marrow smear cytology shows increased numbers of poorly differentiated myeloid precursors and monocytes. Note the paucity of polymorphs and the hypogranular nature of the monocytic cells.

Histologic correlation with the WHO and FAB classifications

There is only a limited correlation between the histologic findings in MDS and the separate categories recognized by the WHO or FAB classifications. In general, a low blast cell count correlates with RA and RARS, whereas with an increase in the number of blast cells the syndrome is more likely to be RAEB or RAEBt. Immunohistochemistry, using CD34, c-kit (CD117) or TdT to highlight blast cells, may be of use in identifying cases of RAEB and RAEBt.[11]

Chronic myelomonocytic leukemia

Clinical features

Clinical features include anemia, hepatosplenomegaly and, occasionally, skin infiltrates. The clinical course is usually protracted although transformation to an acute leukemia may occur.

Diagnosis

The diagnosis is usually made on the marrow aspirate and peripheral blood examination. The peripheral blood monocyte count is $>1 \times 10^9/L$ (of which <5% are blasts). The marrow is hypercellular with <20% blasts. Cytologic examination shows hyperplasia of granulocytic precursors, usually hypogranulated, with poor polymorph differentiation and often also increased numbers of somewhat dysplastic monocytes (Fig. 5.9).

Histopathology of the bone marrow

The appearances seen in most trephines are those of a myeloproliferative disorder and changes indicative of myelodysplasia are usually absent. The cytologic appearances are characteristically those of a leukemic infiltration of the marrow by cells showing a variable differentiation between granulocytes and monocytes (the so-called myelomonocyte) (Fig. 5.10).

Immunocytochemical demonstration of myeloid and monocytic antigens may be helpful in confirming the diagnosis.

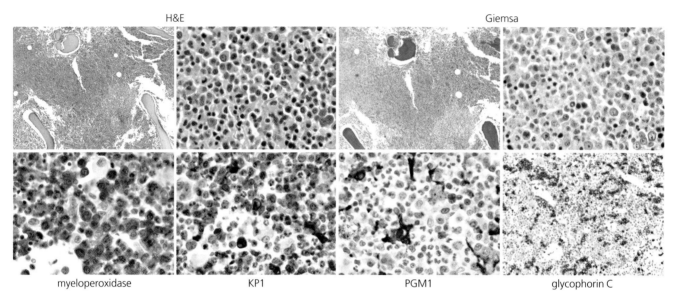

H&E   Giemsa

myeloperoxidase   KP1   PGM1   glycophorin C

Fig. 5.10 In chronic myelomonocytic leukemia (CMML) the marrow is hypercellular and is characterized by an increased number of myelocytes with a lack of more mature granulocytes. Top row: H&E and Giemsa. Bottom row shows the granulocytic precursors (myeloperoxidase) and immature monocytes (KP1 positive, PGM1 negative—these are two CD68 switch variants the latter being absent on immature monocytes and macrophages). Glycophorin C immunostaining outlines the frequently accompanying dyserythropoiesis.

Diagnostic problems

Differential diagnosis

Other diseases can produce a myelodysplastic-syndrome-like picture in the marrow. Hairy cell leukemia and HIV infection are two of the most common examples and have been considered in other chapters.

Distinction between MDS, acute leukemia and aplastic anemia in marrows that are hypocellular is difficult. Another diagnostic problem is the separation of RAEBt and CML in accelerated phase which can only really be separated by examination of the aspirate smears.

Areas such as these can rarely be resolved by histology alone and emphasize the need for close clinical correlations.

Secondary MDS

MDS may follow the use of chemotherapy or radiotherapy, for example in the treatment of Hodgkin lymphoma or myeloma. Secondary MDS, like primary MDS, may progress to AML. The marrow is often hypocellular and dyserythropoiesis is a prominent feature.

Overlap between myelodysplasia and myeloproliferation

In a minority of cases it may not be possible on histologic criteria alone to make a definite diagnosis of myelodysplasia or myeloproliferation. This reflects the fact that there are no absolute histologic features pathognomonic for either condition. Clinical details and cytogenetic studies will only resolve some of these cases. This has led to a view that myelodysplasia and myeloproliferation are a spectrum of myeloid neoplasia rather than separate entities.

References

1 Bennett JM, Catovsky D, Daniel MT, *et al.* The French–American–British (FAB) Co-operation Group. Proposals for the classification of myelodysplastic syndromes. *Br J Haematol* 1982; **51**: 189–99.

2 Jaffe ES, Harris NL, *et al.* (eds) *Pathology and Genetics of Tumours of Haematopoietic and Lymphoid Tissues.* Lyon: IARC Press, 2001.

3 Frisch B, Bartl R. Bone marrow histology in myelodysplastic syndromes. *Scand J Haematol* 1986; **Suppl 45**: 21–37.

4 Fenaux P, Jouet JP, Zandecki M, *et al.* Chronic and subacute myelomonocytic leukaemia in the adult; a report of 60 cases with special reference to prognostic factors. *Br J Haematol* 1987; 65: 101–6.

5 Thiede T, Engquist L, Billstrom R. Application of megakaryocytic morphology in diagnosing 5q– syndrome. *Eur J Haematol* 1988; **41**: 434–7.

6 Verhoef G, De Wolf-Peeters C, Kerim S, *et al.* Update on the prognostic implication of morphology, histology and karyotype in primary myelodysplastic syndromes. *Hematol Pathol* 1991; **5**: 163–75.

7 Tricot G, De Wolf-Peeters C, Vlietinck R, *et al.* Bone marrow histology in myelodysplastic syndromes. *Br J Haematol* 1984; **58**: 217–25.

8 Kitagawa M, Kamiyama R, Takemura T, *et al.* Bone marrow analysis of the myelodysplastic syndromes; histological and immunohistochemical features related to the evolution of overt leukemia. *Virchows Archiv B Cell Pathol* 1989; **57**: 47–53.

9 Delacrétaz F, Schmidt P-M, Piquet D, *et al.* Histopathology of myelodysplastic syndromes. *Am J Clin Pathol* 1987; **87**: 180–6.

10 Rios A, Cañizo C, Sanz MA, *et al.* Bone marrow biopsy in myelodysplastic syndromes; morphological characteristics and contribution to study of prognostic factors. *Br J Haematol* 1990; **75**: 26–33.

11 Horny H-P, Wehrmann M, Schlicker HUH, *et al.* QBEND10 for the diagnosis of myelodysplastic syndromes in routinely processed bone marrow biopsy specimens. *J Clin Pathol* 1995; **48**: 291–4.

Chapter 6 Myeloproliferative disease

Myeloproliferative disease (MPD) is a spectrum of clinical entities characterized by a neoplastic proliferation, believed to arise from a malignant transformation at the marrow stem cell level. Depending on which pathway of differentiation is undertaken by the progenitor cell, a variety of distinctive histologic appearances are produced. These have traditionally been grouped together on the basis of the dominant cell line present in the marrow and the associated peripheral blood picture. Because the defect lies at the level of the stem cell or thereabouts, many cases show features of two or more groups. In addition, the natural course of the disease results in progressive alterations in the histologic appearance with time. The consequences for the histopathologist are that the appearances do not always allow a precise subclassification nor do they always correlate with the clinical features.

Classification of MPD

There are four diseases, well defined clinically, that constitute myeloproliferation:
1 Chronic myeloid leukemia (CML)
2 Polycythemia vera (PV)
3 Essential thrombocythemia (ET)
4 Myelofibrosis (MF)

Chronic myeloid leukemia

Chronic myeloid leukemia (CML) is characterized by the proliferation of differentiated granulocytes. Neoplastic proliferation of erythroid and megakaryocytic members is less obvious. The term CML is synonymous with chronic granulocytic leukemia (CGL), although rarely other forms occur (e.g. chronic eosinophilic, neutrophilic or basophilic leukemia).

The majority of cases (90%) will have the Philadelphia chromosome (Ph) which involves the translocation of the

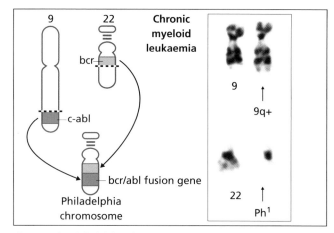

Fig. 6.1 The Philadelphia chromosome.

c-abl proto-oncogene from its site on chromosome 9 to the breakpoint cluster region (BCR) of chromosome 22, usually abbreviated as t(9t;22g-) (Fig. 6.1). Those cases lacking the Philadelphia chromosome (atypical CML) usually possess a genetic rearrangement within the major BCR (M-BCR) on chromosome 22. A small number of cases lack both the Philadelphia chromosome and M-BCR rearrangement, which appears to indicate a poorer prognosis.[1,2] In the three other forms of MPD (polycythemia rubra vera [PRV], ET and MF) the Philadelphia chromosome is absent.

Clinical features

CML is a disease of middle to old age. Clinical features include anemia, tiredness, bruising and, in more advanced stages, splenomegaly and skin infiltrates. The peripheral blood white cell count is raised, typically exceeding 100×10^9/L, of which the majority are neutrophils and myelocytes. Median survival varies considerably from 6 to 55 months.

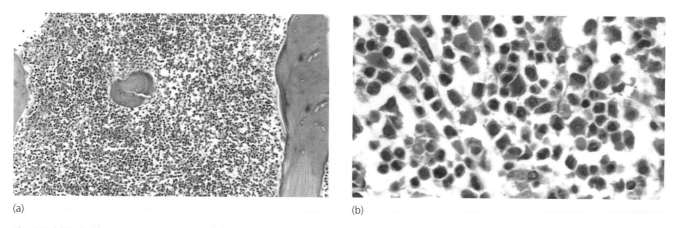

(a)

(b)

Fig. 6.2 (a) Typical low power appearances of chronic myeloid leukemia (CML). Note lack of fat spaces. H&E. (b) High power. Giemsa.

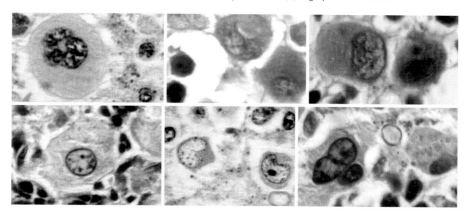

Fig. 6.3 Atypical megakaryocytes in CML. Giemsa.

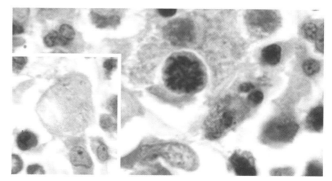

Fig. 6.4 Examples of two pseudo-Gaucher cells in CML. Giemsa.

Histopathology of the bone marrow

The bone marrow is typically hypercellular, showing profound granulocytic differentiation (Fig. 6.2).

Abnormal proliferation in the erythroid and megakaryocytic series is also frequently present although this may be minimal and require careful inspection to detect. The erythroid changes are usually those of immaturity (left-shifting). Megakaryocytes are smaller than normal, increased in number and usually mononuclear (Fig. 6.3).

Cytologic atypia with clustering may be seen but is less marked than in other forms of MPD. The presence of abnormal forms around ectatic sinuses can be helpful in diagnosis, although this is more prominent as a feature of ET.

Macrophages with crystalloid inclusions ("pseudo-Gaucher" cells) (Fig. 6.4) are reported in a significant number of cases. Mast cells, plasma cells and lymphoid cells may also be present in increased numbers as a reactive phenomenon.

An increase in reticulin staining is common, with the presence of severe diffuse reticulin fibrosis being associated with a shorter survival (Fig. 6.5).

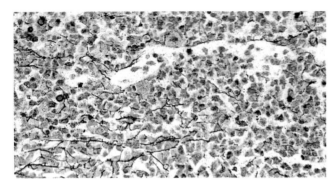

Fig. 6.5 Typical reticulin pattern in CML. Silver stain.

Table 6.1 Histologic features helpful in distinguishing early chronic myeloid leukemia (CML) from leukemoid reaction.

Feature	CML	Leukemoid reaction
Fat cells	Absence of fat cells next to bone trabeculae (i.e. loss of 1st fat space)	Preservation of paratrabecular fat cells
Megakaryocytes	Dwarf forms atypical, mononuclear, small clusters	Normal size or immature, diffuse
Pseudo-Gaucher cells	Present in some cases	Absent in most cases
Hemosiderin	Normal	Increased

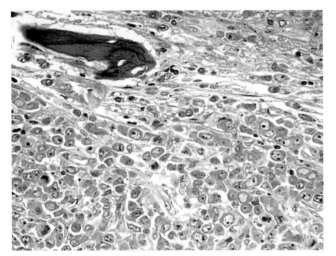
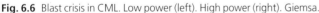
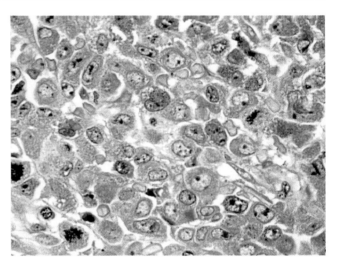

Fig. 6.6 Blast crisis in CML. Low power (left). High power (right). Giemsa.

Diagnostic problems

Two situations present particular diagnostic difficulties.
1 *CML vs. reactive hyperplasia (leukemoid reaction).*
Distinguishing between CML and a highly reactive marrow with an associated leukemoid reaction can be difficult. Causes of such a reaction include infections, cancer outside the marrow, lymphomas particularly Hodgkin lymphoma and autoimmune disease. Examination for the features shown in Table 6.1 may help in making this distinction.

2 *Prediction of impending blast crisis (i.e. transformation to acute leukemia).* CML is a relentless disease progressing towards acute leukemia, usually myeloid. The point of impending transformation cannot be detected by examination of peripheral blood or marrow smears. In the trephine it has been reported that infiltrates of blast cells and promyelocytes 4–8 cells thick in a perivascular and paratrabecular distribution indicates a high probability of transformation to acute leukemia in the ensuing 6 months (Fig. 6.6).[3]

It has also been suggested that increased numbers of CD34 positive cells are predictive of a poorer prognosis.[4]

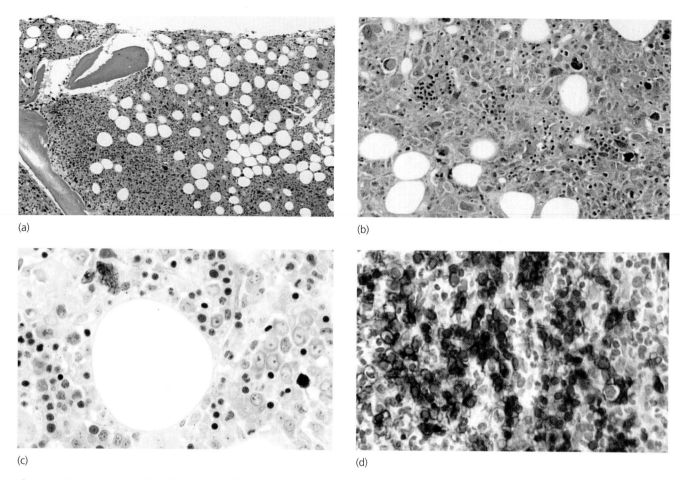

Fig. 6.7 Polycythemia vera (PV). (a) Low power. H&E. (b) Low power. Giemsa. (c) Erythroid differentiation. Giemsa. (d) Confirmed by immunostaining for glycophorin C.

Polycythemia vera

Polycythemia vera (PV) is a neoplastic proliferation with erythroid differentiation resulting in an increased mass of red blood cells. Being a myeloproliferative condition other cell lines are also involved so that an associated increase in granulocytes and platelets is common. Most cases of PV will progress to myelofibrosis (particularly those showing marked megakaryocytic features) with subsequent blast transformation into acute myelocytic leukemia (AML).

The nomenclature of this condition varies and includes polycythemia vera and primary proliferative polycythemia.

Clinical features

The clinical presentation is variable and relates mainly to the patient's polycythemia. Symptoms include headache, dizziness and visual disturbances and may be associated with gout, pruritis or occlusive vascular disease.

Histopathology of the bone marrow

The bone marrow is hypercellular with prominent erythroid differentiation (Fig. 6.7). Florid megakaryocytic proliferation is usually present, many of which are large pleomorphic types often gathered together in prominent clusters (Fig. 6.8).

Large dilated sinuses filled with red blood cells are common (Fig. 6.9) and are usually associated with increased reticulin throughout the marrow (Fig. 6.10). This will in time lead onto the development of an associated fibrosis which usually changes the clinical features to those of myelofibrosis (Fig. 6.11). Reactive plasma cells, macrophages and lymphoid cells (forming nodular aggregates in some cases) are common.

H&E   Giemsa

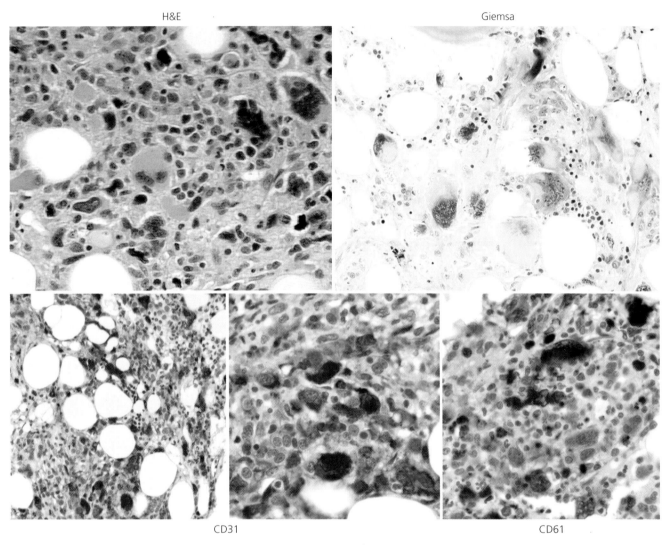

CD31   CD61

Fig. 6.8 Abnormal megakaryocytes in PV. (a) H&E. (b) Giemsa. (c) Immunostains for CD31 and CD61 highlight the megakaryocytes. Note the heterogeneity of the immunostaining which is a feature of the abnormal megakaryocytes in these myeloproliferative disorders.

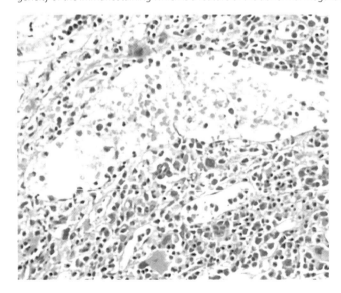

Fig. 6.9 Large dilated sinus in PV. H&E.

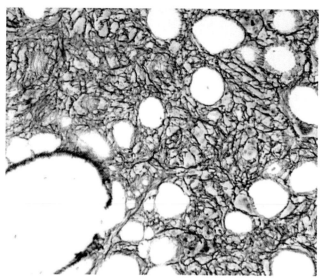

Fig. 6.10 Increased reticulin in PV.

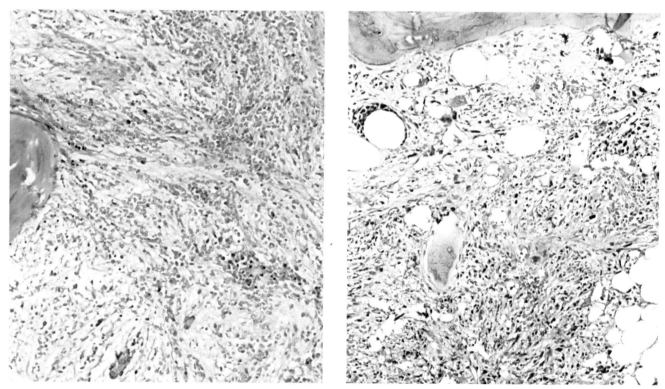

Fig. 6.11 Two cases of PV with associated myelofibrosis. In the first case the clinical pattern was still that of PV whereas the second had developed chronic myelofibrosis (so-called post polycythemic myelofibrosis). Giemsa.

Table 6.2 Histologic features of polycythemia vera (PV) not found in CML.

Erythroid hyperplasia and paratrabecular erythroid islands
No stainable iron (metabolized by the proliferating erythroid cells)
Left-shifted granulopoiesis
Giant megakaryocytes

Diagnostic problems

1 *Distinction between PV and CML with prominent megakaryocytes.* Although these conditions are usually distinguished on clinical grounds, there are a number of histologic features that separate them (Table 6.2).

2 *Distinction between PV and secondary polycythemia.* Cytologic atypia (although admittedly not marked in PV) and abnormal architectural changes are absent in secondary polycythemia. Furthermore, marrow cellularity of more than 75% and loss of the first fat space makes a diagnosis of secondary polycythemia unlikely.

Essential thrombocythemia

In this subgroup of MPD, megakaryocytes are the dominant cell line. They produce large numbers of platelets, which are often functionally impaired.

Clinical features

The disease tends to follow an indolent clinical course, but can transform into acute leukemia. The major clinical features are illustrated in Fig. 6.12.

Histopathology of the bone marrow

The marrow is usually markedly hypercellular. The hallmark is the presence of increased numbers of megakaryocytes. Many are giant forms with marked nuclear atypia (Fig. 6.13).

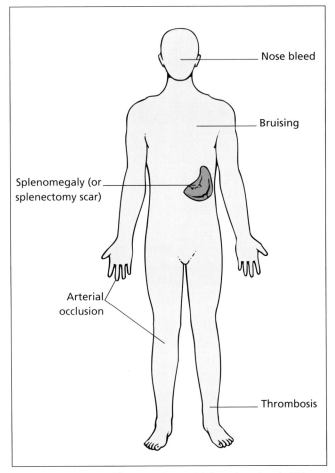

Fig. 6.12 Major clinical features of essential thrombocythemia (ET).

They occur in clusters and often congregate near sinuses into which they disgorge clouds of platelets (Fig. 6.14).

Granulopoiesis and erythropoiesis are usually normal. Fibrosis is usually absent but when it occurs is considered a bad prognostic indicator. This fibrosis reflects increasing dysfunction of the megakaryocytes. This leads to local accumulation of fibrogenic platelet-derived growth factors which would normally be discharged into the circulation (Fig. 6.15).

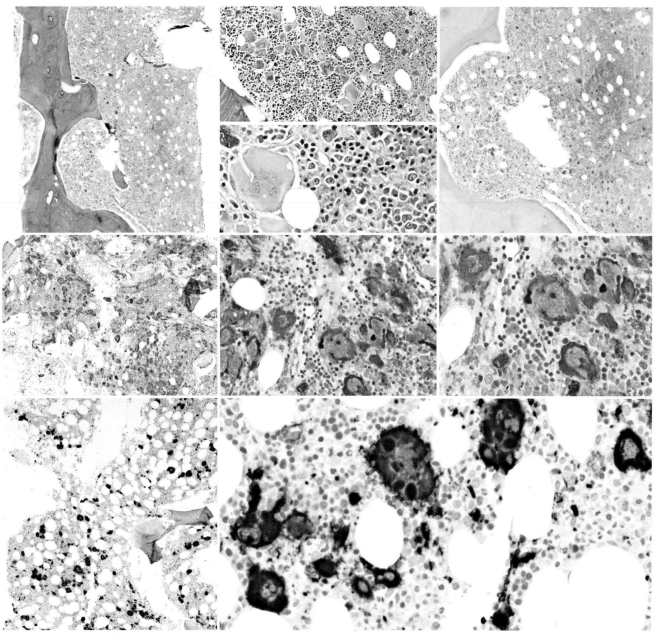

Fig. 6.13 Typical histologic appearances of ET shown by Giemsa (left and centre) and H&E (right) on top row. The abnormal megakaryocytes are highlighted by immunostaining for CD31 (middle row) and CD61 (bottom row). Note in both the high power Giemsa and immunostains that abnormal megaplatelets can be detected within the cytoplasm of the larger megakaryocytes. This is a feature rarely seen in reactive megakaryocytes.

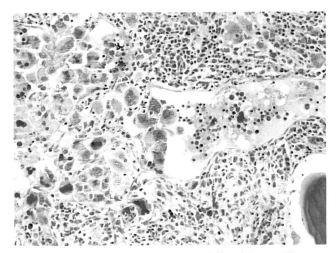

Fig. 6.14 Megakaryocytes clustering around dilated sinuses. Giemsa.

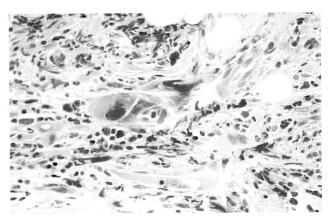

Fig. 6.15 Fibrosis associated with abnormal megakaryocytes in ET. Giemsa.

Diagnostic problems

1 *Philadelphia chromosome positive cases.* Less than 10% of patients with the clinical features of ET have a Philadelphia chromosome. In these patients the marrow histology is more akin to CML (Fig. 6.16). These patients have a worse prognosis, transforming to acute leukemia in 4–7 years.[5] The WHO classification has excluded these cases from the category of ET by definition although without any discussion of the topic. However, these cases are familiar to all clinicians and contin-ue to generate some controversy in the literature.[6] Currently, the pathologist needs to be aware of these cases although they should be categorized as CML if following the current WHO classification.

2 *ET vs. reactive thrombocytosis.* Certain conditions can produce large numbers of megakaryocytes in the bone marrow. A brief list is given in Table 6.3. If fibrosis is also present one should look for evidence of metastatic carcinoma in the marrow because this can produce megakaryocytic hyperplasia which might be misdiagnosed as MPD (Table 6.4).

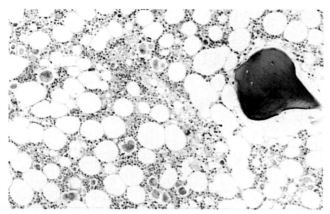

Fig. 6.16 CML-like appearances in Philadelphia chromosome positive case with the clinical features of ET (see text previous page).

Table 6.3 Causes of megakaryocytic hyperplasia.

Post splenectomy
Hemorrhage
Malignancy
Crohn disease
Rheumatoid arthritis
Hepatitis
Iron deficiency
Idiopathic thrombocytopenic purpura (ITP)

Table 6.4 Distinction between essential thrombocythemia (ET) and reactive thrombocytosis.

ET	Reactive thrombocytosis
Megakaryocytes	Megakaryocytes
Giant forms	Normal or small
Clustered	Separate
Paratrabecular	Central
Atypical forms	No atypia
Emperipolesis—occasional	Emperipolesis—common
Erythropoiesis and granulopoiesis are normal	Erythropoiesis and granulopoiesis are right-shifted

Chronic idiopathic myelofibrosis (primary myelofibrosis)

This is probably not a separate entity but represents a response by the marrow to the presence of the neoplastic cells in one of the other forms of MPD. The fibrosis results from fibroblast stimulation by platelet-derived growth factors released by dysfunctional megakaryocytes (Fig. 6.15).

When the fibrosis occurs as the dominant feature in the marrow at presentation it is referred to as chronic idiopathic myelofibrosis. It may then not be possible to identify the abnormalities of a pre-existing subgroup of MPD. PV, ET and CML can all evolve into myelofibrosis. When this progression is clearly documented this is known as secondary myelofibrosis. In practice these conditions are often indistinguishable.

Clinical features

These are summarized in Fig. 6.17.

Histopathology of the bone marrow

The morphology is characterized by well-vascularized fibrosis radiating from endosteal and pericapillary regions (Fig. 6.18). In some cases there is osteoblastic proliferation with new bone formation, often referred to as osteomyelofibrosis (Fig. 6.19). It is nearly always possible to identify abnormal megakaryocytes within this fibrosis although immunostaining may be necessary to confirm their lineage (Fig. 6.19). A thorough search of a myelofibrotic trephine will usually reveal areas of underlying MPD (Fig. 6.20) although it is believed that some cases are entirely primary (also known as agnogenic myelofibrosis).

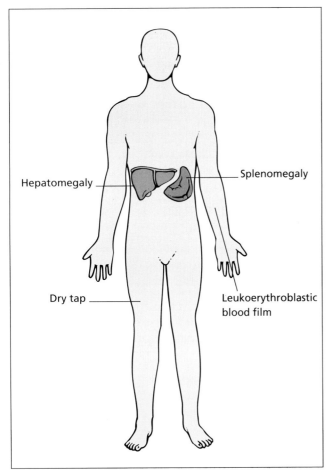

Fig. 6.17 MPD—myelofibrosis.

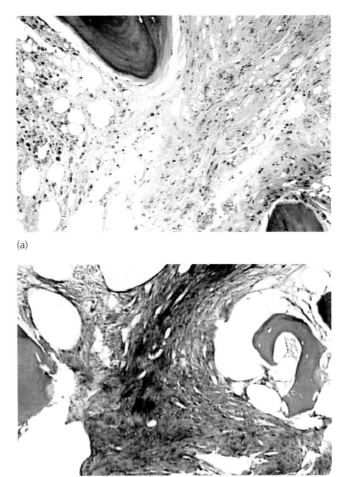

Fig. 6.18 Dense fibrosis in primary myelofibrosis.
(a) Giemsa. (b) Reticulin.

Giemsa

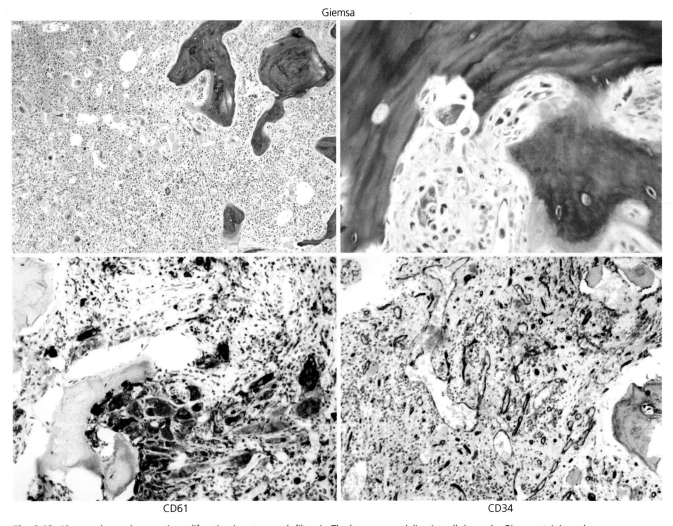

CD61   CD34

Fig. 6.19 Abnormal megakaryocytic proliferation in osteomyelofibrosis. The boney remodeling is well shown by Giemsa staining whereas immunostaining for CD61 (here) or CD31 will be needed to give a clear picture of the megakaryocytes. Note the increased vascularity associated with this condition which is best seen by immunostaining for CD34 in this case.

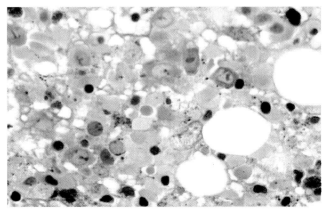

Fig. 6.20 Polycythemia vera (PV) -like area in primary myelofibrosis. Giemsa.

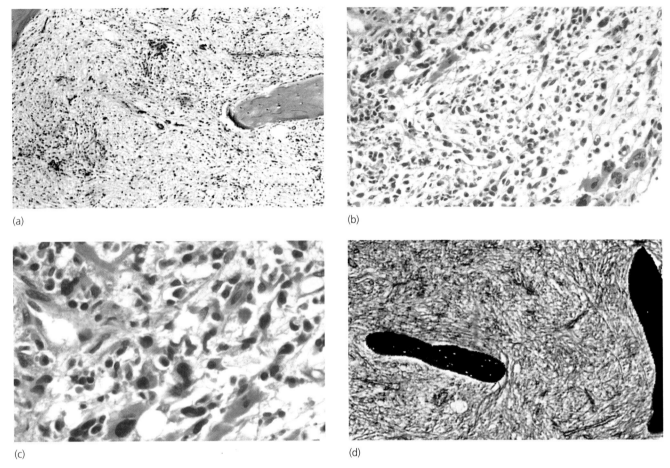

(a)

(b)

(c)

(d)

Fig. 6.21 Acute myelofibrosis (of M7 type). (a–c) H&E. (d) Reticulin.

Acute myelofibrosis

There are two acute fibrotic conditions that have been referred to under this name. The more common is probably acute megakaryoblastic (M7) leukemia without blast cells in the peripheral blood. In the other, which is rare, this relationship is arguable. Here the picture is dominated by pancytopenia and a rapid downhill course without any real evidence of leukemia. The marrow histology is hypocellular with the fat spaces replaced by highly vascular fibrous tissue (Fig. 6.21).[7]

Diagnostic difficulties

Distinction from other forms of fibrosis

A number of other conditions can cause extensive marrow fibrosis and should be considered in the differential diagnosis (Table 6.5).

Distinguishing between MDS and MPD (Table 6.6)

There is no doubt that a number of patients seem to show features, both clinically and histologically, of MDS and MPD. This may reflect imprecision in the current means of classifying these disorders although it is more likely that biologically there is considerable overlap between them. Karyotype analysis is becoming increasingly important in providing more objective criteria.

Table 6.5 Causes of secondary diffuse fibrosis in the bone marrow.

All other myeloproliferations
Acute leukemias other than M7
MDS
Lymphoma:
  both Hodgkin lymphoma and non-Hodgkin lymphoma
Myeloma
Mastocytosis
Carcinoma and sarcoma
TB and other granulomatous disorders
Others including fractures, toxins and irradiation

MDS, myelodysplastic syndrome; TB, tuberculosis.

Table 6.6 Comparison of myelodysplastic syndrome (MDS) with myeolproliferative disease (MPD).

MDS	MPD
Abnormal topography	Normal topography
Immaturity	Usually full maturity
Ineffective hematopoiesis, i.e. 'penias'	Effective hematopoiesis, i.e. 'cytosis'
Stem cell defect reflected as premalignant, i.e. dysplastic changes	Stem cell defect reflected in more obvious malignant changes

Mast cell disease

Neoplastic conditions of mast cells are rare.[8,9] This has resulted in a lack of reliable information on the clinical course and histologic classification. The only entity likely to be encountered in the bone marrow is systemic mastocytosis (SM). This has two forms:

1 *Benign*. This is associated with skin involvement (urticaria pigmentosa) and is rarely associated with myeloproliferative disorders.

2 *Malignant*. This is not associated with urticaria pigmentosa. However, 75% of cases will be associated with MPD with some progress to acute leukemia. Mast cell leukemia is rare.

Histopathology of the bone marrow

The marrow is usually hypercellular (Fig. 6.22) and focally infiltrated by aggregates of mast cells often known as mast cell granulomas. These may have a perivascular and paratrabecular distribution (Fig. 6.23). The infiltrate consists of mast cells, lymphocytes, plasma cells, eosinophils and sea-green histiocytes (Fig. 6.24) surrounding the mast cell precursors in the granulomas. These cells have a bland cytologic appearance, they may be spindled and their nuclei are round or oval and may be indented (Fig. 6.24). The granules may be apparent on H&E but are better appreciated on Giemsa (Fig. 6.25 and 6.26), toluidine blue (Fig. 6.27) or naphthol-AS-D-chloracetate esterase (Leder) stains. Neoplastic mast cells have a characteristic myelomonocytic immunophenotype with the three best immunostains being c-kit[10] (CD117), mast cell tryptase[11] (Fig. 6.27) and CD68 (Figs 6.26 and 6.28).

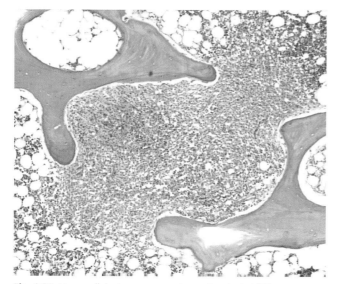

Fig. 6.22 Hypercellular bone marrow in mastocytosis. H&E.

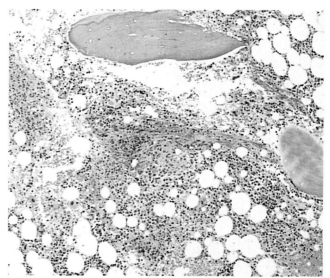

Fig. 6.23 (a)

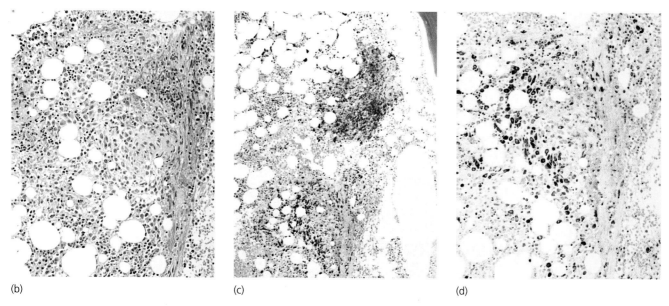

(b)

(c)

(d)

Fig. 6.23 So-called "mast cell granulomas" in systemic mastocytosis. (a,b) H&E. (c,d) Giemsa.

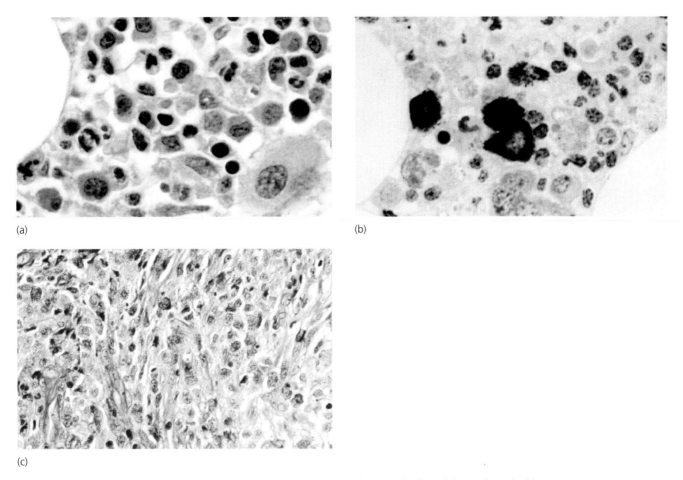

(a)

(b)

(c)

Fig. 6.24 Cytologic appearances of mastocytosis. (a) H&E. (b,c) Giemsa. Note how spindle shaped these cells can be (c).

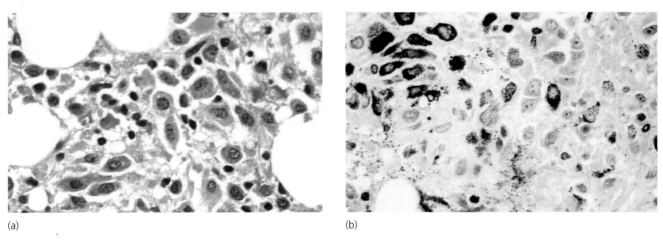

(a)

(b)

Fig. 6.25 Granulation in mast cells. (a) H&E. (b) Giemsa.

Giemsa

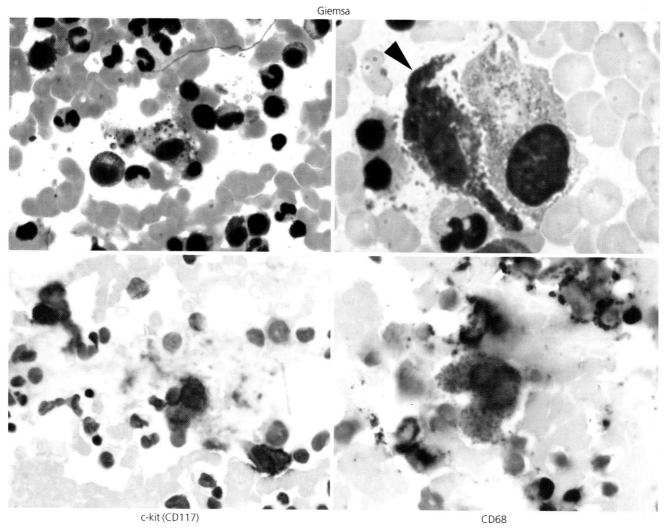

c-kit (CD117)

CD68

Fig. 6.26 Cytologic appearances of systemic mastocytosis showing the atypical mononuclear cells with irregular granulation (next to a mature mast cell in the high power Giemsa [arrowhead] for comparison). These cells are characteristically immunostained for c-kit (CD117) and CD68.

The infiltrate is often associated with fibrosis, an increased number of eosinophils and bone changes which may include osteosclerosis, osteopenia and osteolysis. Some patients have widespread osteoporosis. Distinguishing between the benign and malignant forms histologically is not always possible. In benign SM the mast cells do not show cytologic atypia, the marrow fat is preserved and the infiltrate is nodular rather than diffuse. This contrasts with the malignant form of SM

where the amount of marrow fat is reduced and the mast cells may be atypical, diffusely infiltrative and are likely to be accompanied by the histologic features of MPD. The abnormal expression of CD2 and CD25 on malignant but not reactive mast cells may help with this distinction[12] (Fig. 6.29).

A very uncommon mast cell proliferation known as "eosinophilic histiocytic lesion" appears to involve only the bone marrow and can be histologically indistinguishable from SM.[13]

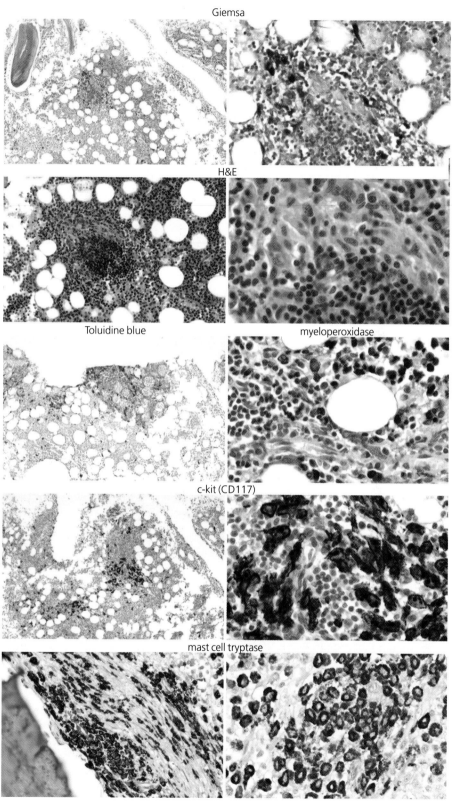

Fig. 6.27 Another typical case of sytemic mastocytosis showing the granuloma formation with Giemsa and H&E. Toluidine blue staining will also identify the mast cells but immunostaining for c-kit (CD117) or mast cell tryptase is far superior. Normal mast cells are myeloperoxidase negative although neoplastic ones may occasionally express it weakly.

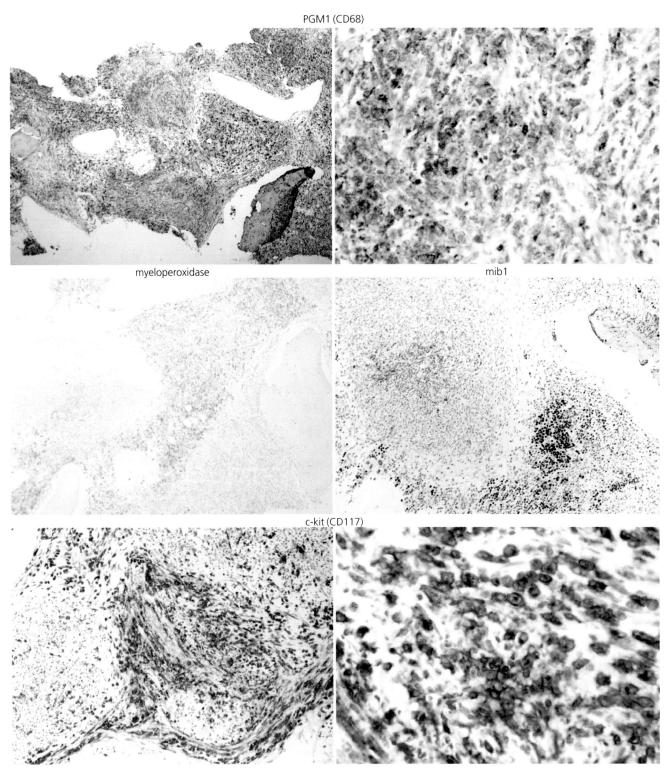

Fig. 6.28 Typical immunostaining of systemic mastocytosis for CD68 (antibody PGM1), myeloperoxidase, mib1 and c-kit (CD117).

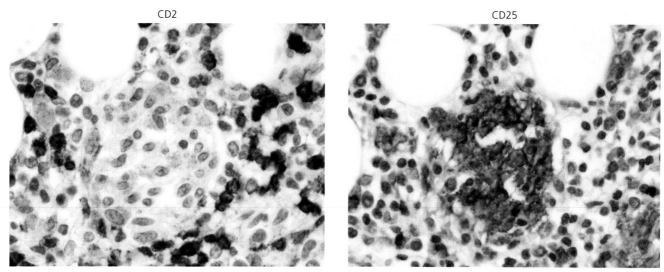

Fig. 6.29 Neoplastic mast cells are positive for CD2 and CD25 which are not present on normal mast cells.

Table 6.7 Immunocytochemical distinction of systemic mastocytosis (SM) and Hodgkin lymphoma (HL).

Antigen	SM	HL
CD30	–	+
CD68	+	–
CD117	+	–
Mast cell tryptase	+	–

Differential diagnosis

The focal pattern of involvement that often occurs in SM may superficially resemble that of Hodgkin lymphoma of the marrow where focal areas of fibrosis are seen. In addition, both entities may contain considerable numbers of eosinophils. However, the presence of large atypical cells with prominent eosinophilic nucleoli (i.e. Hodgkin and Reed–Sternberg cells and/or the appropriate immunocytochemistry) will exclude SM (Table 6.7).

Although most anti-CD68s will show some positivity, it is useful to employ those antibodies (e.g. KP1) recognizing the granulocytic end of the spectrum for stronger, more robust staining of this condition (Fig. 6.26). CD117 and mast cell tryptase are the two other key markers in the diagnosis (Fig. 6.27).

Reactive marrows in HIV-positive patients occasionally show aggregates of fibroblasts, lymphocytes and macrophages, raising a possibility of mast cell disease. Special stains for mast cell granules will be negative.

Transient myeloproliferative disorder

This is a peculiar condition associated with Down syndrome. It occurs in affected neonates with very high white blood cell count, anemia and thrombocytopenia. The marrow has a large population of very primitive blast cells although more normal marrow is also usually present. The blasts are often difficult to type immunocytochemically. Sometimes they are predominantly megakaryocytic but at other times are a mixture of lineages or are unidentifiable (Fig. 6.30). The condition normally resolves of its own accord although some go on to develop AML, which is a risk associated with Down syndrome whether or not the patient has had this transient condition.

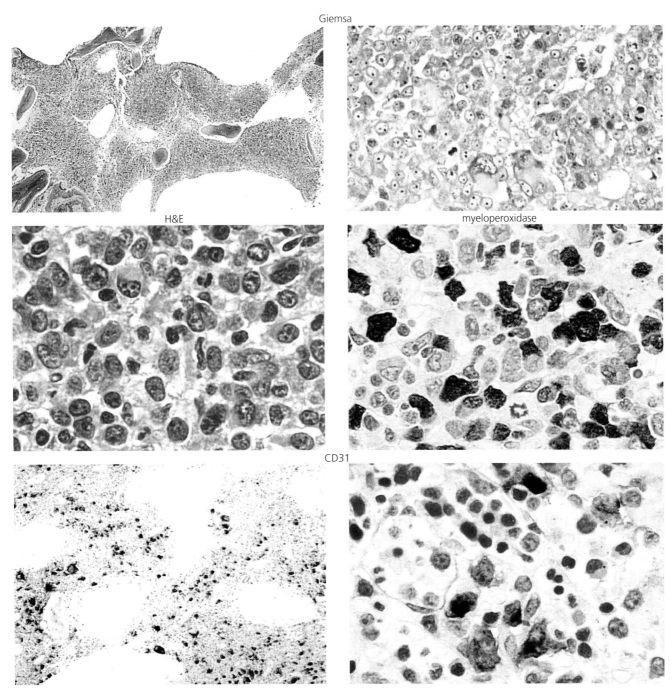

Giemsa

H&E

myeloperoxidase

CD31

Fig. 6.30 A case of transient myeloproliferative disorder in a neonate with Down syndrome. The marrow is hypercellular even allowing for age with a prominent population of primitive blast cells. Some of these can be identified in this case as megakaryocytic (CD31) but others are clearly myeloid (myeloperoxidase). This case resolved after a few weeks and the child has been well for the past 6 years.

References

1 Frisch B, Bartl R, Jaeger K. Histological diagnosis of chronic myelo-proliferative disorders (CMPD). *Hematol Rev* 1989; **3**; 131–47.

2 Martiat P, Michaux JL, Rodhain J. Philadelphia-negative (Ph-) Chronic myeloid leukaemia (CML): comparison with Ph+ CML and chronic myelomonocytic leukaemia. *Blood* 1991; **78**: 205–11.

3 Islam A. Prediction of impending blast cell transformation in chronicgranulocytic leukaemia. *Histopathology* 1988; **12**: 633–9.

4 Orazi A, Neiman R, Cauling H, *et al.* CD34 Immunostaining of bone marrow biopsy specimens is a reliable way to classify the phases of chronic myeloid leukaemia. *Am J Clin Pathol* 1994; **101**: 426–8.

5 Stoll DB, Peterson P, Exten R, *et al.* Clinical presentation and natural history of patients with esssential thrombocythemia and the Philadelphia chromosome. *Am J Hematol* 1991; **27**: 87–97.

6 Fadilah SA, Cheong SK. BCR-ABL positive essential thrombocythaemia: a variant of chronic myelogerous leukaemia or a distinct clinical entity: a special case report. *Singapore Med J* 2000; **41**: 595–8.

7 Hruban RH, Kuhajda FP, Mann RB. Acute myelofibrosis. Immuno-histochemical study of four cases and comparison with acute megakaryocytic leukaemia. *Am J Clin Pathol* 1987; **88**: 578–88.

8 Horny H-P, Parwaresch MR, Lennert K. Bone marrow findings in systemic mastocytosis. *Hum Pathol* 1985; **16**: 808–14.

9 Lennert K, Parwaresch MR. Mast cells and mast cell neoplasia: a review. *Histopathology* 1979; **3**: 349–65.

10 Natkunam Y, Rouse RV. Utility of paraffin section immunostaining for c-kit (CD117) in the differential diagnosis of systemic mast cell disease involving the bone marrow. *Am J Surg Pathol* 2000; **24**: 81–91.

11 Horny HP, Sillaber C, Menke D, *et al.* Diagnostic value of immunostaining for tryptase in patients with mastocytosis. *Am J Surg Pathol* 1998; **22**: 1132–40.

12 Jaffe ES, Harris NL, *et al.* (eds) *Pathology and Genetics of Tumours of Haematopoietic and Lymphoid Tissues.* Lyon, IARC Press: 2001.

13 Rywlin AM, Hoffman EP, Ortega RS. Eosinophilic fibrohistiocytic lesion of bone marrow. A distinctive new morphological finding, probably related to drug hypersensitivity. *Blood* 1972; **40**: 464–72.

Chapter 7 Acute leukemia

There are two main types of acute leukemia: myeloid (AML) and lymphoblastic (ALL). Acute leukemias are blastic proliferations of white cells that usually but not invariably involve the peripheral blood. The exact definition of particular subtypes is often arbitrary (defined by committee consensus) and much unnecessary confusion between histologist and hematologist/oncologist can be avoided by comparing specimens and relating findings to individual patients. This is especially the case when dealing with the overlap between lymphoma and leukemia.

Both acute leukemias affect all ages although their frequencies are quite different. AML is primarily an adult disease with the incidence rising with age whereas more than 85% of cases of ALL are in children aged under 15 years. The prognosis in ALL in children is excellent whereas in AML it is generally poor, particularly in the elderly. Some studies give those over 55 years only a 2% chance of 5-year survival regardless of therapy.

Classification

Since the first edition of this text there has been a major change in the classification of acute myeloid leukemia. The French–American–British (FAB) group classification which had achieved wide acceptance for both AML and ALL[1,2] was based solely on cytologic appearances. It has become increasingly recognized that this is not adequate for clinical purposes and that the underlying cytogenetic abnormalities must also be considered. The clinical importance of these changes cannot be overemphasized and they have been incorporated into the WHO classification published in 2001 where full details can be obtained by the interested reader. AML is now divided into four major groups:

1 AML with recurrent genetic abnormalities: t(8;21), inv(16), 11q23 and t(15;17)
2 AML with multilineage dysplasia
3 AML, therapy related
4 AML not otherwise categorized

Acute myeloid leukemia

Classification

From the point of view of the pathologist these changes have very little effect. Indeed the chapter in the WHO book makes only passing references to histology in all of these categories. Basically, in the first three categories the histology is remarkably similar as we commented previously for the FAB classification. If one is lucky, histology might recognize the t(15;17) promyelocytic leukemias and significant associated dysplastic changes can help recognize category 2. Otherwise the best we can do is identify lineage differentiation in category 4 as monocytic, erythroid or megakaryocytic, just as we did previously for the FAB classification.

Histopathology and immunophenotyping

Acute myeloid leukemia

Another important difference between the WHO classification and the FAB system is that the blast cell count necessary for a diagnosis of AML is reduced from 30% to 20%. The essential contribution of the pathologist is to recognize the blasts as myeloid not lymphoid and to give an estimate of their percentage and distribution. There is no definitive immunophenotype for AML as it is an extremely heterogeneous condition but most cases in WHO categories 1–3 will be myeloperoxidase positive and negative for B and T cell markers. There are some exceptions to this as CD2, CD7 and CD9 can be detected in some cases but provided they are myeloperoxidase positive a diagnosis of AML should be made. Exceptions to this rule are those rare primitive AMLs previously labeled M0 which lack most antigens although with luck will be terminal deoxynucleotidyl transferase (TdT) positive (Fig. 7.1). Other helpful markers are TdT (more commonly positive on ALL though), c-kit (CD117), CD34 and CD56 (Fig. 7.2). Acute promyelocytic leukemia is difficult to detect histologically

CD34 myeloperoxidase

proliferation TdT

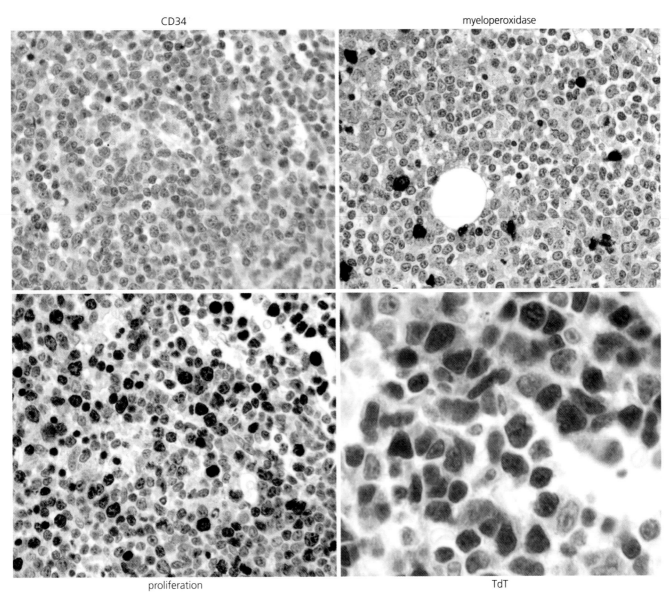

Fig. 7.1 Primitive case of acute myeloid leukemia (AML) positive only for terminal deoxynucleotidyl transferase (TdT).

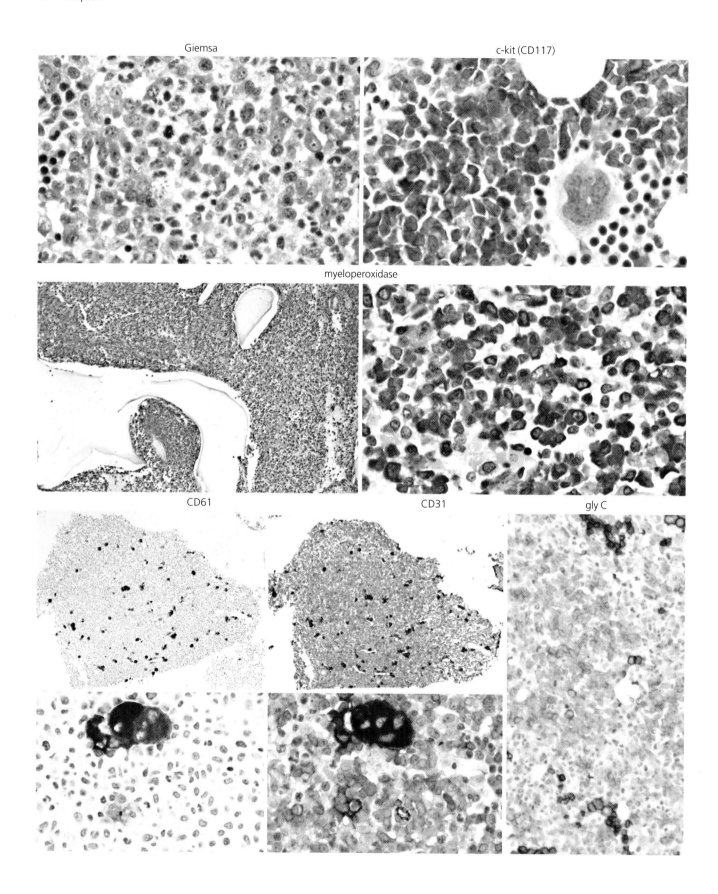

Giemsa

c-kit (CD117)

myeloperoxidase

CD61

CD31

gly C

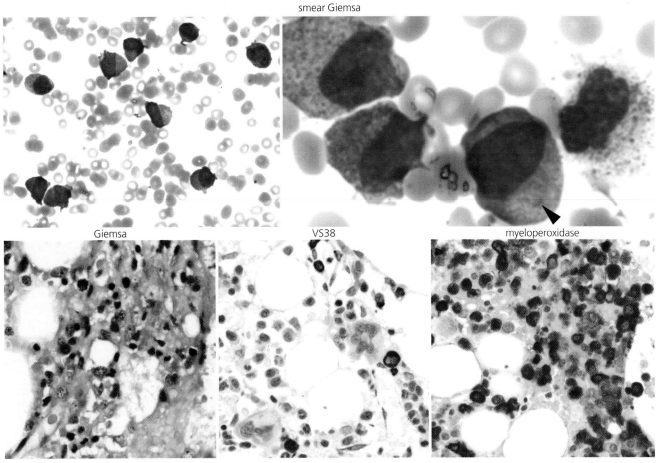

smear Giemsa

Giemsa   VS38   myeloperoxidase

Fig. 7.3 Acute promyelocytic leukemia with abnormal granulated promyelocytes being plentiful in the marrow smear. Note an Auer rod (arrowhead) in the high power. The histology can be confusing at times. This case has a lymphoplasmacytic appearance but is negative for plasma cell markers (VS38) and other lymphoid antigens but positive for myeloperoxidase.

and careful liaison with the hematologists or inspection of the smears in needed (Fig. 7.3). Antibodies recognizing the PML gene product patterns, which would be very helpful, are still not available for use on paraffin sections.

Occasionally AML is sufficiently patchily distributed throughout the marrow that a confident diagnosis cannot be made on cytology alone and here histology provides essential information for the clinician (Fig. 7.4). Category 2 AML (i.e.

that arising with or from myelodysplasia) is important to recognize as it has a poor prognosis. While this information is usually known by the clinicians, histology can highlight this quite successfully in many cases (Fig. 7.5). Finally, there will always be odd cases that have unusual immunophenotypes which require careful clinical correlation so as not to misdiagnose AML as lymphoma or vice versa (Fig. 7.6).

Fig. 7.2 (opposite) Typical case of AML positive for myeloperoxidase and c-kit (CD117). Note for interest the weak positivity for CD31 which is not lineage specific and glycophorin C; such so-called anomalous findings are common in AML.

myeloperoxidase

CD34

CD56

c-kit (CD117)

Giemsa

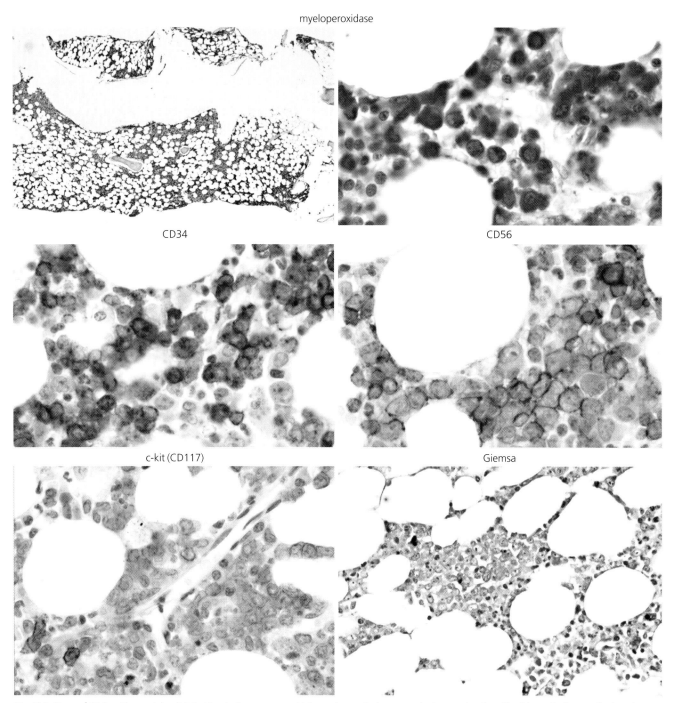

Fig. 7.4 Case of AML with a patchy distribution in the marrow which was inconclusive on aspirate examination. The biopsy is diagnostic showing large numbers of blasts immunostaining for myeloperoxidase, CD34, CD56 and c-kit (CD117).

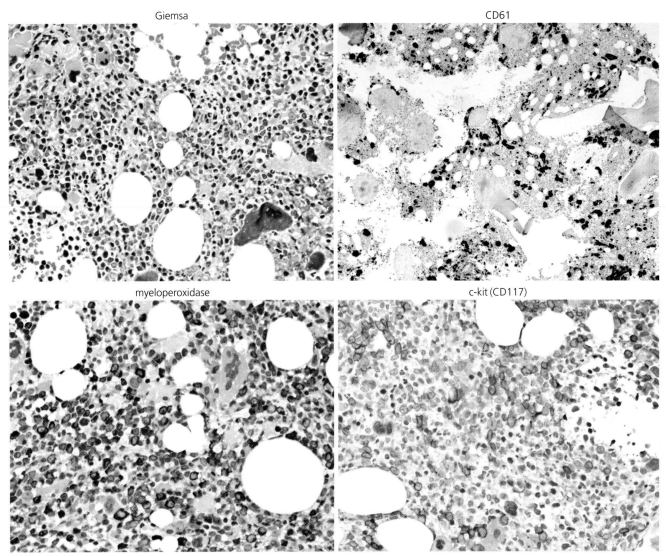

Fig. 7.5 AML arising from a dysplastic marrow (well demonstrated by the megakaryoctic pattern with CD61). Myeloperoxidase and c-kit (CD117) immunostains outline the substantial blast cell population.

Therapy related AMLs can be extremely difficult to diagnose as they are often mixed up with dysplastic marrow elements which represent regenerative changes as much as true myelodysplasia. Careful immunophenotyping and, if possible, comparison with the underlying condition that was treated will usually sort out the true diagnosis (Fig. 7.7). Of course it should never be forgotten that at the same time as a secondary AML arises the previous condition itself may also relapse (Fig. 7.8).

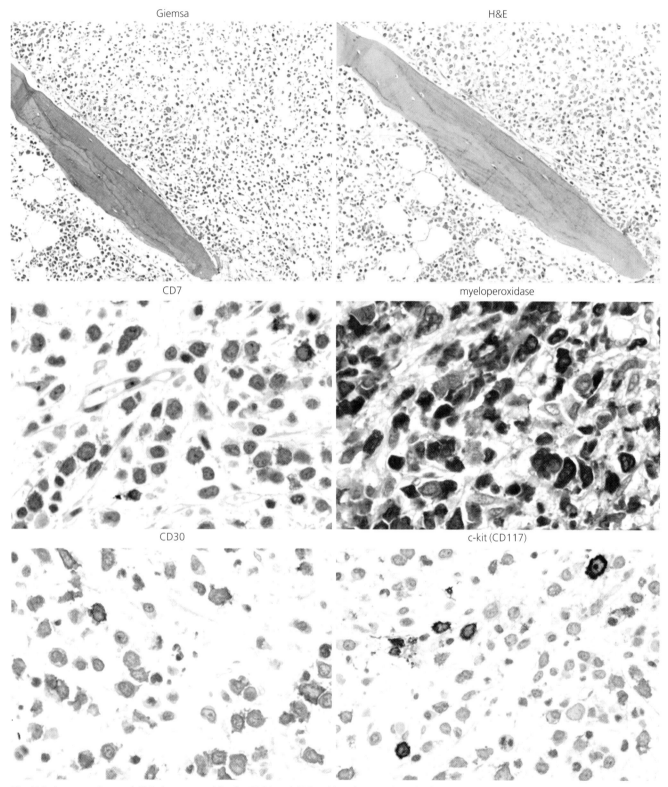

Fig. 7.6 An unusual case of AML that was positive for CD30 and CD7, raising the question whether it was lymphoid in origin. Myeloperoxidase and to a lesser extent c-kit (CD117) positivity on the blasts reveals its true nature.

Secondary AML

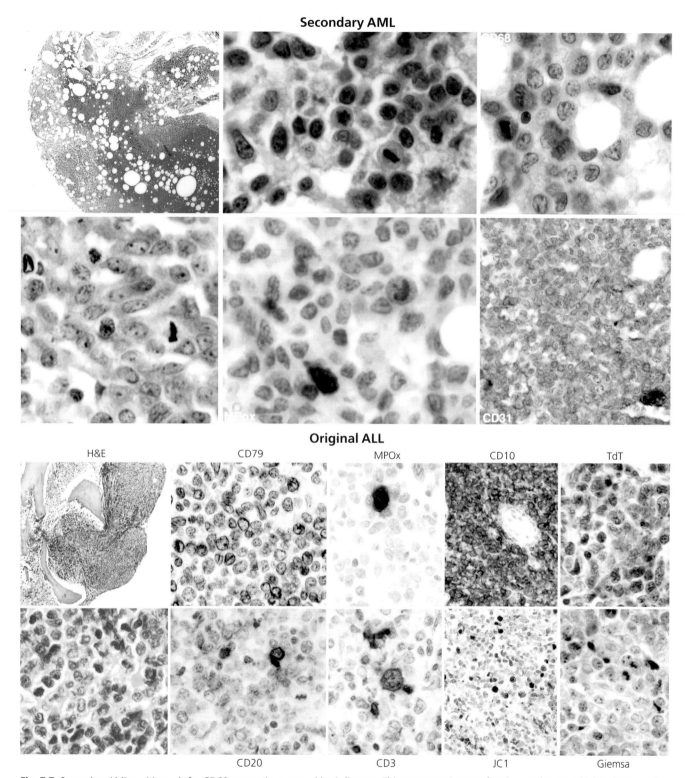

Original ALL

H&E CD79 MPOx CD10 TdT

CD20 CD3 JC1 Giemsa

Fig. 7.7 Secondary AML positive only for CD68 suggesting a monoblastic lineage. This case arose 2 years after therapy for ALL which is shown at the bottom of the figure and has an entirely different immunophenotpye.

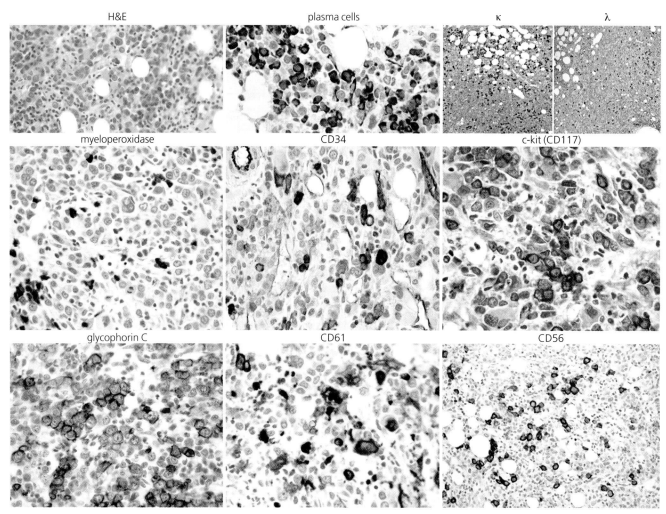

Fig. 7.8 Secondary AML arising 5 years after treatment for myeloma. The AML, although negative for myeloperoxidase, is identified by staining for c-kit (CD117), CD56, CD34, glycophorin C and CD61. As well as this complex AML there is also present a relapse of the myeloma demonstrated by staining for VS38 and light chains (κ and λ).

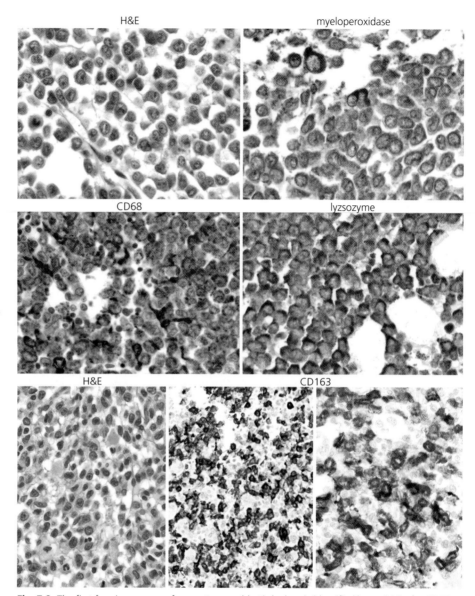

Fig. 7.9 The first four images are of an acute monoblastic leukemia identified by positivity for CD68 and lysozyme. Most cases are negative for myeloperoxidase although this one shows that exceptions occur. The second case (bottom three images) illustrates the value of CD163 in highlighting infiltration by monoblastic leukemia.

Myelomonocytic and monoblastic leukemias

These are important AML subtypes to recognize as they frequently lack myeloperoxidase. In these cases monocytic markers, especially CD68, CD163 and lysozyme, are very important in reaching the diagnosis. Monoblastic leukemia in particular can be confusing as it often presents with extramedullary masses, causing suspicions of lymphoma to be raised (Fig. 7.9).

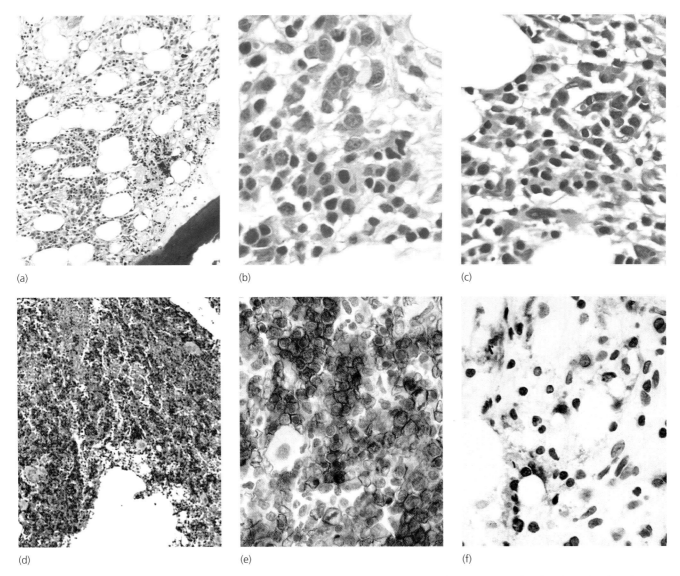

Fig. 7.10 M6 erythroleukemia. The histology is shown in (a,b) Giemsa and (c) H&E. The majority of the cells are erythroid as shown by glycophorin C staining (d,e) but many abnormal cells express other lineage markers such as the megakaryocytic antigen CD61 (f).

Erythroleukemia M6

This is a rare category which it is easy to overlook as myelodysplasia with excess blasts, indeed the borderline between these two conditions is quite uncertain. The erythroid element is predominantly associated with dysplastic erythroid colonies whereas the lineage of most of the true leukemic blasts is uncertain (Fig. 7.10). In cases of doubtful lineage it is probably better to categorize them as AML rather than force a diagnosis of erythroleukemia.

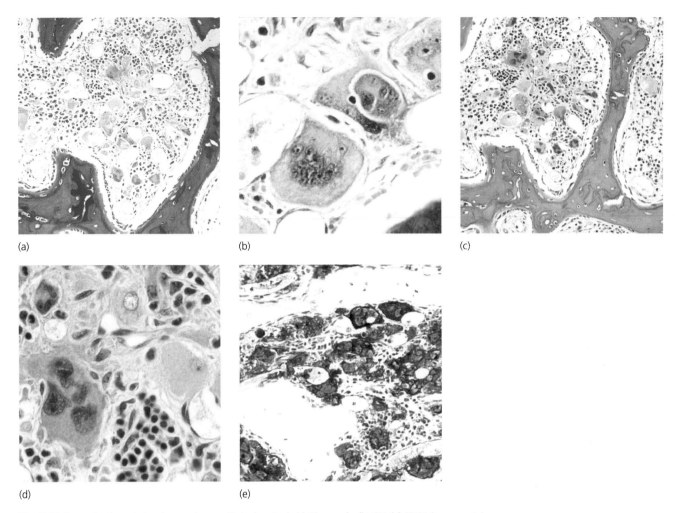

Fig. 7.11 Example of an obviously megakaryocytic leukemia. (a,b) Giemsa. (c,d) H&E. (e) CD31 immunostain.

Megakaryoblastic and megakaryocytic leukemia M7

This acute leukemia has a variable morphology from the recognizably megakaryocytic to the frankly bizarre where it can be identified only on the basis of immunocytochemistry. As mentioned in Chapter 6 on myeloproliferative diseases, many cases of acute myelofibrosis are examples of M7 leukemia (Fig. 7.11).

Hypoplastic AML

These patients present with pancytopenia and a "dry tap" on aspiration. Aplastic anemia is usually the main differential, although leukemia is often suspected clinically due to a few suspicious blast-like cells being seen in the peripheral blood. The trephine usually makes the diagnosis by showing discrete collections of primitive blast cells in an otherwise empty marrow. It is said that hypocellular AML should be distinguished from hypocellular myelodysplastic syndrome (MDS). It is common to find evidence of both conditions so that distinguishing hypocellular AML from refractory anemia with excess blasts is not always easy. AML should not be diagnosed unless more than 20% of the cells can be clearly identified as blast cells (Fig. 7.12).

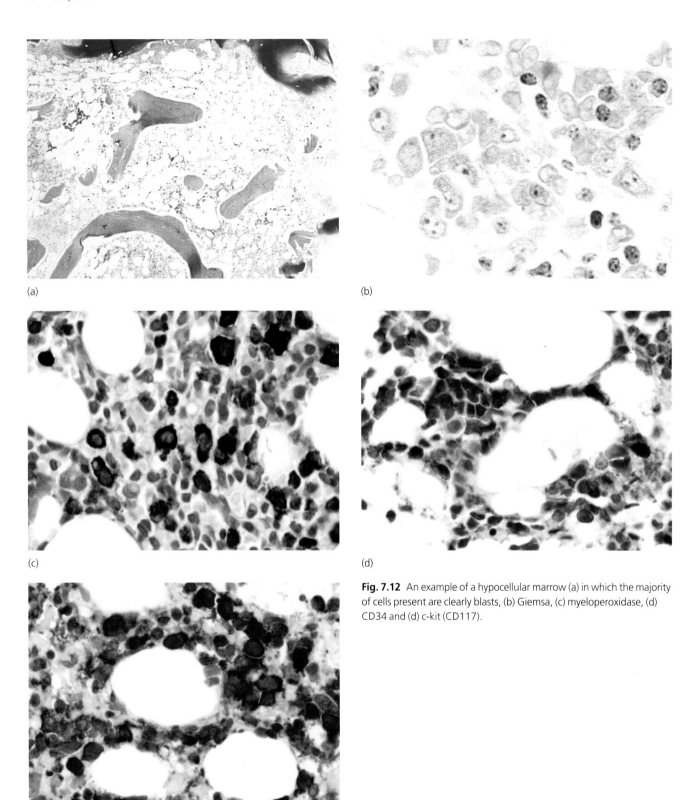

(a)

(b)

(c)

(d)

(e)

Fig. 7.12 An example of a hypocellular marrow (a) in which the majority of cells present are clearly blasts, (b) Giemsa, (c) myeloperoxidase, (d) CD34 and (d) c-kit (CD117).

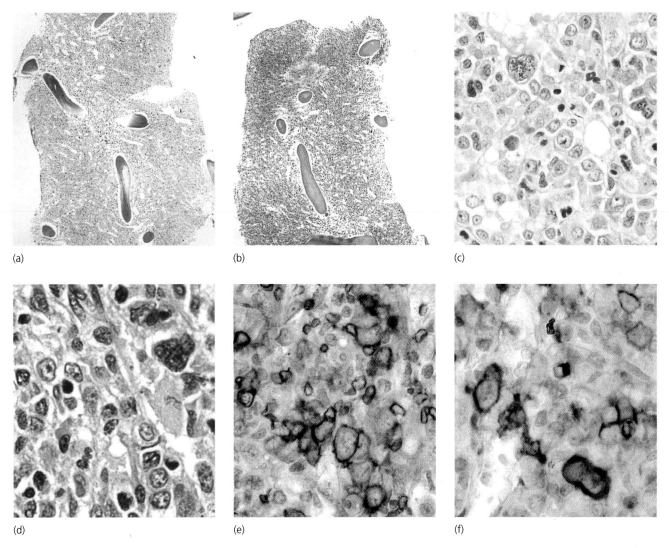

Fig. 7.13 Hypercellular marrow (a,b) packed with abnormal pleomorphic blasts (c,d), some expressing erythroid (e) and others megakaryocytic (f) antigens. (a,c) Giemsa. (b,d) H&E. (e,f) Immunoperoxidase.

Diagnostic problems

Unclassifiable cases

Leukemia is no different to most other tumor classifications with cases showing overlapping features. In the case of AML the histologist will probably not become involved in disputes over M0–M5 but occasional bizarre cases spanning M6 and M7 do occur (Fig. 7.13). In the current state of knowledge such cases do not influence therapeutic decision making.

AML or ALL

It is frequently difficult to decide on histologic grounds whether an acute leukemia is lymphoid or myeloid. Careful immunophenotyping as detailed in this chapter for AML and in Chapter 8.2 will usually resolve any difficulties (Fig. 7.14).

In some cases the pathologist needs to be cautious not to overlook those biphenotypic leukemias that express both lymphoid and myeloid markers. Fortunately, these cases are uncommon and often arise as a pre-existing leukemia relapses or transforms so that the therapeutic options are currently limited. Nevertheless, close liaison with clinical hematologists will usually result in an acceptable conclusion especially if there is a clear cytogenetic phenotype such as t(9;22) or 11q23 abnormalities, both changes known to span myeloid and lymphoid differentiation.

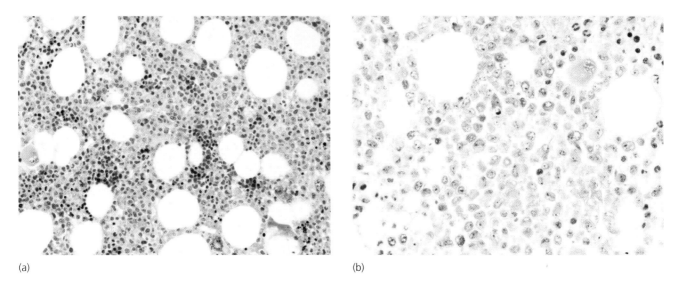

(a)

(b)

Fig. 7.14 Case of ALL initially believed to be AML on cytologic and histologic grounds. (a) Giemsa. It was negative for all myeloid markers but expressed CD79a, a B cell antigen (b), as well as other ALL markers such as CD10.

(a)

(b)

Fig. 7.15 Marrow biopsy from a patient treated with granulocyte colony-stimulating factor (GCSF) for neutropenia subsequent to chemotherapy for myeloma. This patient did not develop AML and returned to normal hematologic parameters some time afterwards.

Growth factors

The increasing use of growth factors, especially granulocyte colony-stimulating factor (GCSF), to assist patients with neutropenia after chemotherapy may cause considerable problems in marrow histology as it causes a significant increase in myeloid blast activity and can easily be mistaken for AML (Fig. 7.15). This conundrum can be completely baffling if there is evidence clinically of relapse of an underlying myeloid leukemia whose treatment has involved GCSF administration (Fig. 7.16).

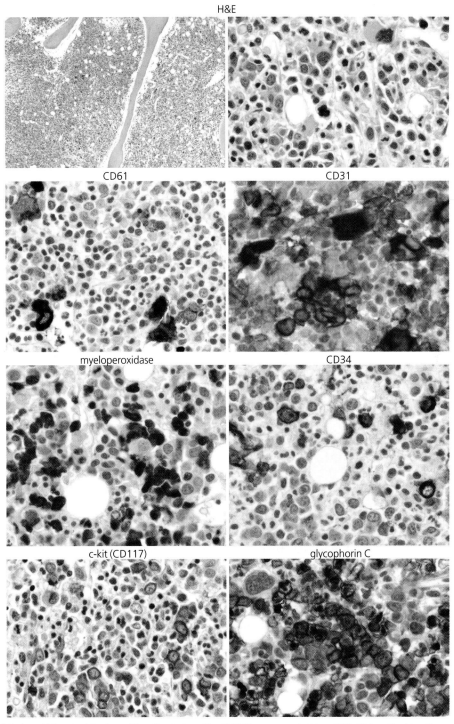

Fig. 7.16 This case illustrates the difficulty of distinguishing the blastic proliferation induced by GCSF from an underlying AML. This patient had been treated for acute megakaryoblastic leukemia with chemotherapy and GCSF. The patient became pancytopenic and blasts with complex cytogenetic abnormalities were identified. Immunophenotyping shows a complex picture suspicious of AML (e.g. c-kit [CD117] positive blasts) but not diagnostic. The patient relapsed with frank AML some weeks later.

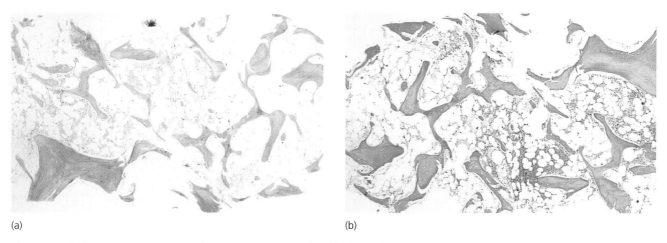

(a)   (b)

Fig. 7.17 Typical empty marrow seen a week or so after transplantation. (a) Giemsa. (b) H&E.

Acute lymphoblastic leukemia

Reflecting the histologic bias of the authors, a full presentation of this topic will be found in the chapter on lymphoma.

Transplantation and graft-versus-host disease

The place of bone marrow transplantation in the treatment of both hematologic and other malignancies is still not fully established. Many, if not most procedures, remain experimental, so close liaison with appropriate clinicians is essential in the interpretation of bone marrow and other histology from these patients. Three approaches are currently in use employing allografts, autografts and peripheral stem cell rescue. All of these employ prior intensive chemotherapy so that initial bone marrow samples are characterized by severe hypocellularity (Fig. 7.17).

The marrow regeneration is usually led by erythropoiesis followed by megakaryocytic and granulocytic proliferation (Fig. 7.18). Without too many complications the marrow regenerates steadily to produce relatively normal indices in the peripheral blood over a period of a few months. During this period the regenerating colonies can appear profoundly dysplastic which should not be misinterpreted as a recurrence of tumor (Fig. 7.19). Relapse of a leukemia or lymphoma can occur at any time even after several years and is typically dramatic (Fig. 7.20).

An early complication is failed or slow regeneration. These are being treated with a number of recombinant growth factors that themselves can produce dysplastic or bizarre appearances. Infectious complications are unfortunately common and include viral, fungal and mycobacterial diseases whose appearances are the same as those seen in other immunocompromised individuals.

The hematopathologist is often asked to diagnose acute graft-versus-host disease in skin or rectal biopsies of allograft patients. When severe the diagnosis is clinically obvious but mild cases are indistinguishable from drug-induced changes and only careful clinical review can separate these. There is now a growing consensus that mild graft-versus-host disease in allografted patients is beneficial because of an associated graft versus leukemia or lymphoma reaction (Fig. 7.21). As always, clinical correlation is necessary because immunosuppressive drugs can give an effect identical to that seen with graft-versus-host disease (Fig. 7.22).

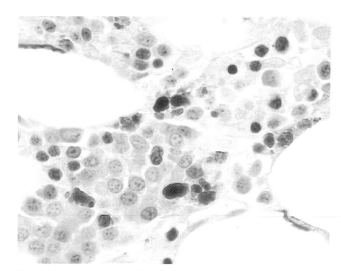

Fig. 7.18 Regenerating erythroid colonies approximately 1 month after engraftment.

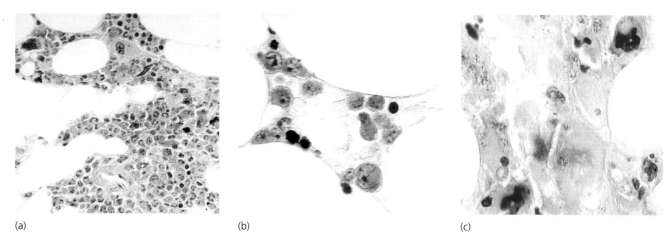

(a)   (b)   (c)

Fig. 7.19 Relatively normal cellularity a few months after engraftment. (a) Giemsa, but note the dysplastic erythroid cells. (b) Giemsa and megakary-ocytes. (c) Giemsa, which should not be confused with leukemic relapse.

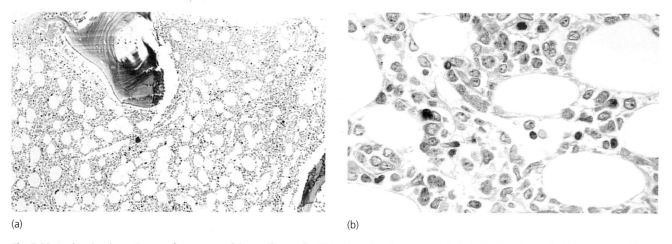

(a)   (b)

Fig. 7.20 Leukemic relapse 6 years after a successful engraftment for AML. Note that the marrow is full of primitive blast cells. (a) Low power. (b) High power. Both Giemsa.

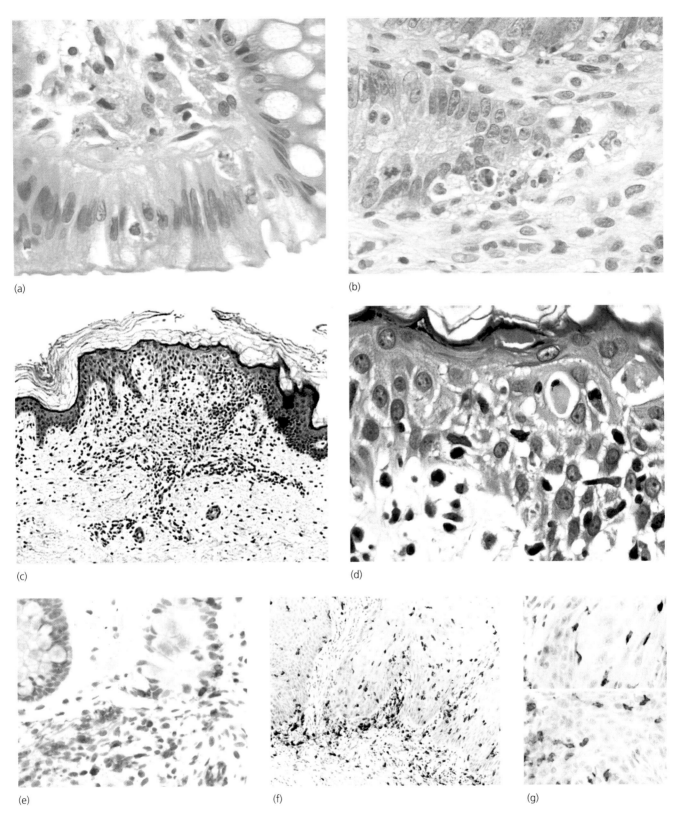

Fig. 7.21 Typical graft-versus-host disease in a bone marrow allograft recipient. (a,b) Show mild and severe involvement of rectal mucosa and (c,d) illustrate severe skin disease at low and high power. Immunostaining will highlight the infiltrating lymphocytes as T cells of CD8 subtype (e–g).

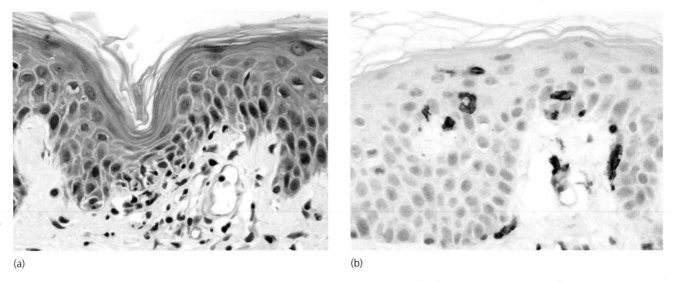

(a)

(b)

Fig. 7.22 Skin biopsy from a bone marrow transplant recipient showing all of the features of graft-versus-host disease as noted in Fig. 7.21. This patient did not have clinical disease and after modification of the immunosuppresive regimen it remitted.

References

1 Bennett JM, Catovsky D, Daniel MT, *et al.* Proposals for the classification of the acute leukaemias (FAB cooperative group). *Br J Haematol* 1976; **33**: 451–8.

2 Bennett JM, Catovsky D, Daniel MT, *et al.* Proposed revised criteria for the classification of acute myeloid leukaemia. *Ann Intern Med* 1985; **103**: 626–9.

Chapter 8.1 Lymphomas

There can be few areas of histopathology encountered by the general surgical pathologist that produce such a "heart sink" feeling as lymphoma classification. The apparent difficulty with lymphoma classification has been partly brought about by the genuine complexity of the subject, with the constant need to update classifications in the light of scientific advances, and partly by the existence of a number of influential pathologists, many with strong personalities, who have actively promoted their own classifications in an atmosphere that was more competitive than cooperative. However, the confusion of multiple classifications is now largely resolved by the work of the International Lymphoma Study Group which formulated the Revised European and American Lymphoma (REAL) classification[1] which has now largely been incorporated into the World Health Organization (WHO) classification[2] which has found universal acceptance as the established lymphoma classification.

The historical perspective outlining the development of lymphoma classification is shown in Table 8.1. No classification exists that is perfect but in the final analysis the purpose of a classification is to provide clinically relevant information in terms of prognosis and predicting behavior and in determining the most effective therapeutic regimens. It should be understandable, reproducible and based on concepts that have scientific credibility.

What does the clinician require from the pathologist?

The clinician will need to know the following so that the appropriate therapy can be given:
1 Is it Hodgkin or non-Hodgkin lymphoma?
2 If it is Hodgkin lymphoma, which subtype?
3 If it is non-Hodgkin lymphoma, what is the subtype and is it likely to be high or low grade?
4 Is there histologic evidence of marrow involvement?

The following chapters discuss a variety of lymphomas selected from the latest WHO classification of lymphomas and they are presented largely in that format. We regard them as representing the lymphomas most likely to be encountered by the general surgical pathologist. Some of the more frequently encountered entities are described in greater detail. The WHO classification has also brought in some linguistic changes to terminology which are not discussed in the text. Hodgkin's disease becomes Hodgkin lymphoma, non-Hodgkin's lymphoma becomes non-Hodgkin lymphoma and Burkitt's lymphoma is Burkitt lymphoma. These changes are not fundamentally significant. They grate on some but are lapped up by others and it is our view that readers should use whichever they prefer. In this text to prevent repetition we have adopted the WHO terminology (reluctantly for at least one of us!).

Those lymphomas to be discussed are as follow:
1 *Non-Hodgkin lymphoma*

B cell	Lymphoblastic
	Chronic lymphocytic leukemia
	Lymphoplasmacytic/immunocytoma
	Mantle cell
	Follicular
	Marginal zone
	Hairy cell
	Multiple myeloma
	Diffuse large B cell
	Burkitt
T cell	Lymphoblastic
	Lymphocytic
	Primary cutaneous, i.e. mycosis fungoides/Sézary syndrome
	Large granular lymphocyte
	Peripheral, unspecified
	Angioimmunoblastic
	Adult T cell
	Anaplastic large cell

2 *Hodgkin lymphoma*
Classic subtypes
- nodular sclerosis
- mixed cellularity
- lymphocyte rich

Lymphocyte predominance

Table 8.1 Historical perspective of the development of lymphoma classification.

1870s Concept of malignant lymphoma originated by Billroth

1890s Recognition of Hodgkin lymphoma and non-Hodgkin lymphomas as separate disease groups by Dreschfeld and Kundrat

1900–1950 Awareness of different groups within the non-Hodgkin lymphomas but the terminology used was not standardized and certain terms meant different things to different pathologists (e.g. lymphosarcoma, reticulum cell sarcoma)

1960s Emergence of the first clinically useful classifications in terms of providing prognostic information. These were the Rappaport classification for non-Hodgkin lymphoma and the Lukes–Butler classification for Hodgkin lymphoma. Rappaport classified lymphomas primarily on the growth pattern (i.e. nodular or diffuse) and also placed some weight on the degree of differentiation and morphologic similarity of the malignant cell compared with either normal small lymphocytes or histiocytes (hence the erroneous term "histiocytic lymphoma"; these lymphoma cells are now known to be transformed lymphocytes)

1970s Increasing knowledge of the functional and morphologic heterogeneity of the immune system (e.g. T and B cells) led to modification of Rappaport's classification to recognize additional specific entities (e.g. Burkitt and lymphoblastic lymphoma)

1975 Increased recognition by hematopathologists of the large number of morphologically different lymphoid cells within normal lymphoid tissue led to classifications based on detailed morphologic descriptions of lymphoid cells. The front runners of this type of classification were, in Europe Professor Lennert's Kiel classification and in the USA the Lukes–Collins classification. Both attempted to postulate an origin for various lymphomas from normal cells within lymph nodes (e.g. follicular lymphoma cells had their normal counterpart in germinal centers of secondary lymphoid follicles). Around the same time a number of others produced similar classifications also largely based on the appearance of the malignant cells

1980s The large number of classifications at this time created much confusion and frustration amongst clinicians. This prompted the National Cancer Institute to facilitate the development of a working formulation for clinical usage. This was to serve as a "Rosetta stone" for lymphoma classifications allowing translation of one classification's terminology into another's. Although it was not intended as a classification it became one for many pathologists and clinicians, particularly in the USA

1990 The Kiel classification was updated to take account of advances in immunology and molecular genetics; it included a classification of T cell lymphomas. The major emphasis was still on the morphologic detail of the lymphoma cells as revealed by the Giemsa stain. The preference in the USA and the UK for hematoxylin and eosin stain partly limited the use of this classification in these countries. Many felt that the subtle nuances in cytologic detail described by Lennert were beyond the average jobbing surgical pathologist. As one delegate declared during debate at an international lymphoma meeting, "We don't all have Lennert's eyes."

1995 The Revised European and American Lymphoma (REAL) classification was proposed by the 19 members of the International Lymphoma Study Group as a consensus classification which draws on the best of current classifications, in particular the Kiel classification, but also incorporates and emphasizes other facets in lymphoma diagnosis (e.g. immunophenotype, genetics and clinical features). In so doing, it moved away from the concept of lymphomas belonging strictly to low or high grade groups and emphasized the heterogeneity of clinical behavior within specific lymphoma types (e.g. not all follicular lymphomas have an indolent clinical course). Lymphomas should be viewed as having a range of possible differentiations in the same way as neoplasms of other tissues. The REAL classification, unlike others, has incorporated Hodgkin lymphoma and attempted to clarify the different subtypes using the same format that it applied to the non-Hodgkin lymphomas .The WHO classification is based on the principles defined in the "Revised European–American Classification of Lymphoid Neoplasms (REAL) classification"…It incorporates input from additional experts in order to update and broaden the consensus on the lymphoid neoplasms, and extends the principles of disease definition and consensus-building to the classification of myeloid, mast cell and histiocytic neoplasms. Over 50 pathologists from around the world were involved in the project. …Thus, this classification represents the first true world-wide consensus classification of hematologic malignancies

The future As our knowledge of lymphomas increases, particularly at a molecular level, new classifications will be developed with more relevance to therapy and prognosis. Pathologists and clinicians must resign themselves to further change in lymphoma classification.

Table 8.2 WHO classification of B cell lymphoma. This list excludes rare subtypes.

Precursor B cell neoplasms
Precursor B lymphoblastic leukemia/lymphoma

Peripheral B cell neoplasms
Chronic lymphocytic leukemia/small lymphocytic lymphoma
B cell prolymphocytic leukemia
Lymphoplasmacytic lymphoma
Mantle cell lymphoma
Follicular lymphoma
Marginal zone B cell lymphoma (nodal, extranodal, splenic)
Hairy cell leukemia
Plasmacytoma/plasma cell myeloma
Diffuse large B cell lymphoma
Burkitt lymphoma

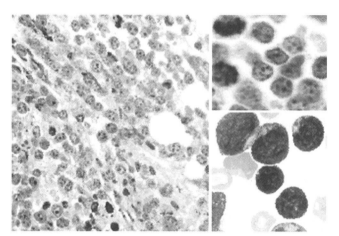

Fig. 8.1 B lymphoblastic leukemia/lymphoma.

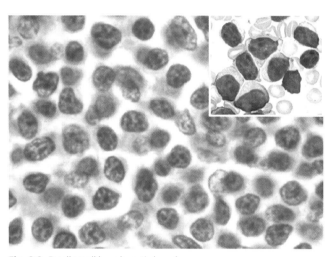

Fig. 8.2 B cell small lymphocytic lymphoma.

World Health Organization classification

Table 8.2 provides a brief overview of the WHO classification of lymphoma.

B cell neoplasms in the WHO classification

The WHO classification focuses attention on non-Hodgkin lymphoma although it also covers Hodgkin lymphoma. The non-Hodgkin lymphomas of B lymphoid origin are divided into those arising from immature cells and those representing more mature B cells.

Precursor B cell neoplasm

B lymphoblastic leukemia/lymphoma. Lymphoblastic neoplasms of B cell type usually present as a leukemia (Fig. 8.1). They typically express markers, such as terminal deoxynucleotidyl transferase (TdT) and CD10, found on early B cells. CD79a (cytoplasmic) and PAX5 (nuclear) are of value because they are often the only B cell markers expressed by these cells that are detectable in paraffin embedded tissue.

Although bone marrow and blood involvement is very common, a few cases are localized as solid tumors, usually in lymph nodes.

The disease, although aggressive, can be cured, particularly when it occurs in children.

Mature B cell neoplasms

B cell small lymphocytic lymphoma (chronic lymphocytic leukemia). Neoplasms composed of small lymphocytes may present as lymphomas or leukemias (Fig. 8.2). The leukemias comprise both chronic lymphocytic and prolymphocytic leukemia. Histologically, small lymphocytic neoplasms show a monotonous infiltration of small cells, but clusters of larger cells ("pseudofollicles or proliferation centers") are a common feature. Occasionally, the neoplastic cells may differentiate to the plasma cell stage but this should not prompt a diagnosis of lymphoplasmacytic lymphoma (Fig. 8.4). Small lymphocytic neoplasms usually express CD5 and CD23, in addition to "pan-B cell" markers. They tend to follow an indolent course.

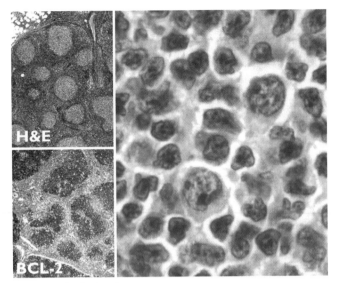

Fig. 8.3 Follicular lymphoma.

Fig. 8.4 Immunocytoma/lymphoplasmacytic lymphoma.

Follicular lymphoma

Follicular lymphoma (Fig. 8.3) constitutes, at least in the West, one of the most frequent non-Hodgkin lymphomas and it is clear that they are the neoplastic equivalent of normal germinal centers. This origin explains their title in the Kiel scheme of "centroblastic/centrocytic" lymphoma. They are usually easy to recognize because of their follicular growth pattern. They occasionally transform into diffuse tumors containing numerous large cells (centroblasts), and then fall into the group of "large B cell lymphoma." The (14;18) chromosomal translocation, present in over 90% of cases, juxtaposes the *bcl2* gene to the immunoglobulin (Ig) heavy chain gene, and this is accompanied by expression of bcl2 protein. This is in contrast to normal germinal center B cells, which are bcl2 negative. Follicular lymphomas that lack this translocation usually also express bcl2 protein and show identical clinical behavior to translocation positive cases. The disease is usually only slowly progressive but is essentially incurable with a significant number of patients finally undergoing transformation to a diffuse large B cell lymphoma.

Lymphoplasmacytic lymphoma (immunocytoma/Waldenström macroglobulinemia)

The neoplastic cell in lymphoplasmacytic lymphoma (Fig. 8.4) is a B lymphocyte, which shows a tendency to differentiate towards the plasma cell stage. IgM is detectable in the cells with plasmacytic features, within the cytoplasm or as intranuclear inclusions (Dutcher bodies). IgM may also appear in the serum as a paraprotein, and the patient may show the manifestations of Waldenström macroglobulinemia. Strong cytoplasmic IgM positivity can help to distinguish the disease from small lymphocytic neoplasms, as does the absence of CD5. The disease is normally indolent but may transform to an aggressive large cell lymphoma. Other B cell neoplasms (e.g. small lymphocytic lymphoma and MALT lymphoma) may show plasmacytoid differentiation so that a diagnosis of lymphoplasmacytic lymphoma should only be made in cases lacking features of other neoplasms.

Mantle cell lymphoma

Mantle cell lymphoma (Fig. 8.5) is equivalent to "centrocytic lymphoma" in the Kiel scheme. This change of name reflects the lack of evidence that the neoplastic cells derive from a germinal center cell (as the term "centrocytic" implies), and the realization that they have many of the features of mantle zone lymphocytes.

The disease usually presents with lymphadenopathy, but may be found at extranodal sites, notably the gastrointestinal tract (lymphomatous polyposis). The neoplastic cells are usually small to medium sized and may have irregular or "cleaved" nuclei, or a more "blastic" appearance. The growth pattern is often nodular and the neoplastic cells tend to "home" to the mantle zones of lymphoid follicles. The malignant cells typically express CD5 and nuclear cyclin D1.

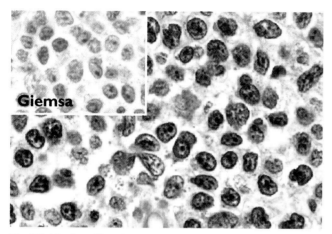

Fig. 8.5 Mantle cell lymphoma.

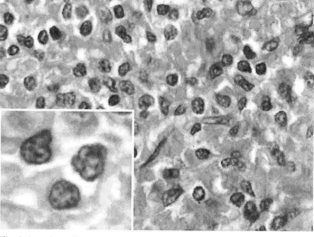

Fig. 8.6 Hairy cell leukemia.

Hairy cell leukemia

Hairy cell leukemia (Fig. 8.6) is characterized by cells with fine villous surface projections (particularly with phase contrast microscopy) and bean-shaped nuclei which are seen in the circulation, the bone marrow and the red pulp of the spleen. The latter sites of involvement account for the pancytopenia and marked splenomegaly. Lymph node infiltration is rare. The cells express, in addition to typical B cell antigens, the receptor for interleukin 2 (CD25) and the CD103 integrin (a cell adhesion molecule). In paraffin sections a distinctive pattern of markers can be detected, and these may be of diagnostic value (e.g. when the marrow shows a low level of infiltration). In addition to pan-B markers such as CD20 and CD79, neoplastic cells express CD68 (as cytoplasmic dots), tartrate resistant acid phosphatase (TRAP) and are labeled by antibody DBA.44. The disease tends to follow an indolent course.

Extranodal marginal zone B cell lymphoma (MALT lymphoma)

Extranodal marginal zone lymphomas (Fig. 8.7) are thought to represent the neoplastic equivalent of the marginal zone cells found in the spleen and lymph nodes in non-nodal sites. These arise typically in the gastrointestinal tract or other extranodal sites, usually glandular epithelial tissues, and are commonly referred to as "MALT lymphomas." MALT stands for mucosa associated lymphoid tissue. These neoplasms derive from the B cells associated with epithelial tissues, and usually arise against a background of reactive lymphoid tissue, in which non-neoplastic germinal centers are prominent. They tend to remain localized, so that their prognosis is usually good, but they can transform to a diffuse large B cell lym-

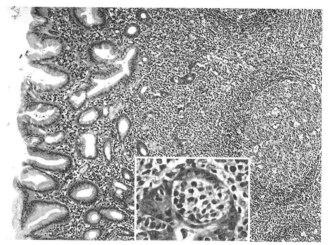

Fig. 8.7 Marginal zone B cell lymphoma, extranodal (MALT-type).

phoma. When they spread to local lymph nodes the MALT lymphoma cells invade the marginal zone and expand the interfollicular region, and some of the lymphoma cells may have a "monocytoid" appearance.

Splenic marginal zone lymphoma

Splenic marginal zone lymphoma (Fig. 8.8) differs from marginal zone lymphoma of MALT type in having a high incidence of bone marrow disease at presentation. It is a rare disease. When lymphoma cells are found in the blood it corresponds to the disease recognized by hematologists as "splenic lymphoma with villous lymphocytes."

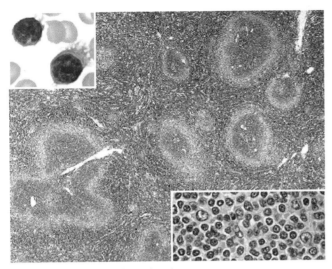

Fig. 8.8 Splenic marginal zone lymphoma.

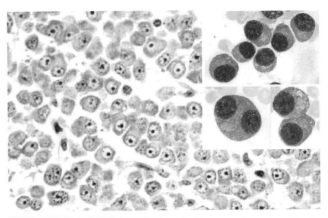

Fig. 8.9 Plasmacytoma/plasma cell myeloma.

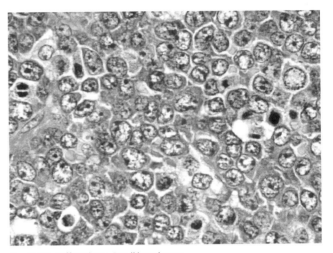

Fig. 8.10 Diffuse large B cell lymphoma.

Plasmacytoma/plasma cell myeloma

Plasma cells are the cells characteristic of myeloma or plasmacytoma (Fig. 8.9), the former term being used when the neoplasm is found in the bone marrow, causing skeletal destruction, and the latter for those rare tumors that arise in soft tissue and other sites. B cell surface antigens are generally absent, in keeping with their loss by normal mature plasma cells, but cytoplasmic Ig (of a single light chain type) is present, accompanied in about 50% of cases by CD79a, one of the two chains of the molecule associated with Ig in B cells. The chromosome abnormality characteristic of mantle cell lymphoma (the (11;14) translocation) is found in some cases. Patients with multiple myeloma usually respond initially to therapy, but almost all relapse after a period of remission.

Diffuse large B cell lymphoma

"Diffuse large B cell lymphoma" (Fig. 8.10) combines the "centroblastic" with the "immunoblastic" category of previous classifications. It is one of the most common categories of non-Hodgkin lymphoma. Pan-B cell markers are expressed, and in a minority of cases the (14;18) chromosomal translocation is present, suggesting an origin from follicular lymphoma in at least some cases. The disease usually requires aggressive treatment, but may respond well, at least for a period.

Primary mediastinal (thymic) lymphoma is a rare subtype of diffuse large B cell lymphoma. The neoplastic cells often have characteristic pale cytoplasm and are thought to arise from intrathymic B cells. Sclerosis is commonly seen and this lymphoma has distinctive clinical features (e.g. it tends to occur in younger female patients and to relapse at extranodal sites).

Burkitt lymphoma

Burkitt lymphoma (Fig. 8.11) was originally described in African patients. The tumor is typically made up of medium sized B cells with a very high proliferation fraction, interspersed with macrophages containing cellular debris, giving the characteristic "starry sky" appearance. The atypical variant may be difficult to distinguish with certainty from diffuse large cell lymphoma. Its B cell phenotype with lack of bcl2 but positivity for CD10 and bcl6 has prompted suggestions that it derives from germinal center cells. In most of these "endemic" African cases Epstein–Barr (EB) viral DNA is found in the malignant cells. Histologically and phenotypically identical cases are also seen in the West. These may arise in patients with AIDS, and the EB virus is also detectable in almost half of these cases. Non-African "sporadic" cases also arise in the absence of immune impairment and EB virus is detectable in less than one-quarter of these cases. Almost all cases, from whatever country, show a chromosomal translocation involving the *myc* gene on chromosome 8 and the gene for Ig heavy chain or, less commonly, one of the two Ig light chain genes. The disease usually responds to aggressive therapy.

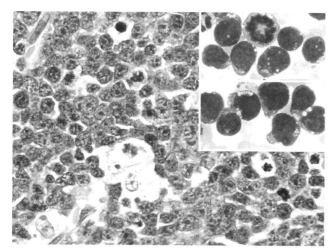

Fig. 8.11 Burkitt lymphoma.

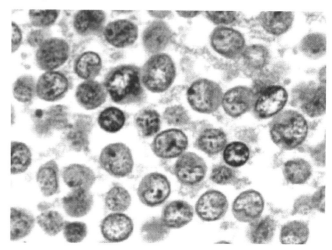

Fig. 8.12 T lymphoblastic leukemia/lymphoma.

Table 8.3 WHO classification of T cell neoplasms

Precursor T cell neoplasms
Lymphoblastic leukemia/lymphoma

Peripheral T cell and NK cell neoplasms
T cell prolymphocytic leukemia
T cell large granular lymphocytic leukemia (LGL)
Mycosis fungoides/Sézary syndrome
Peripheral T cell lymphomas, unspecified
Angioimmunoblastic T cell lymphoma (AILT)
Extranodal NK/T cell lymphoma, nasal type
Enteropathy type T cell lymphoma
Adult T cell leukemia/lymphoma (ATL/L)
Anaplastic large cell lymphoma (ALCL)

NK, natural killer.

T cell and natural killer cell neoplasms in the WHO classification

The other major category of lymphoid neoplasia in the WHO scheme (apart from Hodgkin lymphoma) comprises those arising from T cell or natural killer (NK) cells (Table 8.3). As in the case of the B cell disorders, they are subdivided into lymphoblastic neoplasms, which arise from immature cells of thymic origin, and those that arise from mature peripheral T cells.

T lymphoblastic leukemia/lymphoma

The morphology of lymphoblastic neoplasms of precursor T cell origin is usually indistinguishable from that of B cell lymphoblastic neoplasms (Fig. 8.12). They typically present as acute leukemias but occasionally give rise to tumors in the lymph node or thymus. T cell antigens are present although CD3 is usually, because of the immaturity of the cells, only found in the cytoplasm. The disease is potentially curable with aggressive therapy.

T cell chronic prolymphocytic leukemia (Fig. 8.13)

T cell lymphomas of small lymphocytes resemble small lymphocytic B cell neoplasms in that they often involve the peripheral blood, and their morphology is similar. Generally, their nucleoli are more prominent and the cytoplasm more abundant, so that the cells are classified hematologically as "prolymphocytes." Unlike small lymphocytic B cell lymphoma, pseudofollicles containing larger cells are not seen. These lymphomas express pan-T cell antigens and also CD7, and are commonly CD4 positive. The disease tends to follow a rather more aggressive course than small lymphocytic B cell tumors.

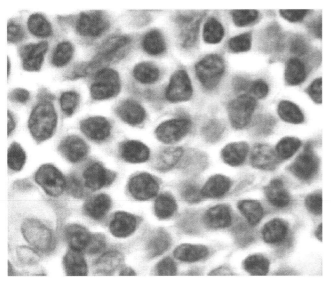

Fig. 8.13 T cell chronic prolymphocytic leukemia.

Peripheral T cell lymphoma, unspecified

The REAL scheme created a single category of "peripheral T cell lymphoma" (Fig. 8.14) because of the lack of reproducibility amongst pathologists of the subtypes recognized by the Kiel classification. The word "unspecified" was added to indicate that it may comprise a number of different entities. This category has been retained in the WHO classification.

These neoplasms typically contain a mixture of small and large neoplastic cells, often with irregular nuclei. There may be a marked infiltration of non-neoplastic cells, including macrophages and eosinophils. In some cases, clusters of epithelioid histiocytes, characteristic of so-called "Lennert" or lymphoepithelioid T cell lymphoma, are seen. A variety of patterns of T cell antigen expression are found, CD4 being more frequent than CD8. Peripheral T cell lymphomas are for some reason seen with greater frequency in the Far East than in Europe and the USA, where they account for less than 20% of non-Hodgkin lymphomas. The prognosis is very variable (although typically poor).

T cell large granular lymphocyte leukemia

Neoplasms arising from "large granular lymphocytes" present most frequently as a hematologic disorder, in which "Tγ lymphocytosis" is associated with neutropenia (Fig. 8.15). A proportion of patients have clinical features of rheumatoid arthritis, and an unclear relationship exists with cases of Felty syndrome. They can be subdivided, on the basis of phenotype, into those that arise from T cells and those that derive from NK cells.

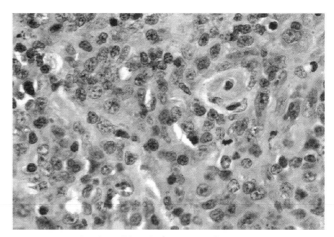

Fig. 8.14 Peripheral T cell lymphoma, unspecified.

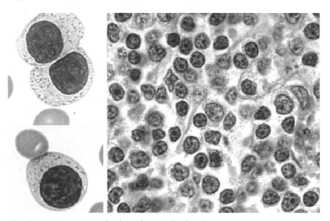

Fig. 8.15 Large granular lymphocyte leukemia.

The disease is usually indolent, although the course tends to be more aggressive in Asian cases, in which the neoplastic cells are of NK type and contain EB viral DNA. The borderline is not always clear between these Asian cases and extranodal NK/T cell lymphomas, nasal type.

Mycosis fungoides/Sézary syndrome

Mycosis fungoides is a T cell lymphoma arising in the skin, but which is referred to as Sézary syndrome when the lymphoma cells are also found in the circulation (Fig. 8.16). The neoplastic cells accumulate in the epidermis, where they may form localized pockets referred to as "Pautrier's microabscesses," and have a typical highly convoluted cerebriform nuclear morphology. As the disease progresses it can spread to lymph nodes, where the interfollicular zones are infiltrated. The cells express pan-T cell antigens, apart from CD7, and are almost always of CD4 or "helper" subtype. The disease follows a variable course but may become widespread and has a tendency to transform to a large cell tumor.

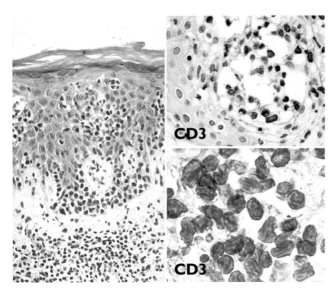

Fig. 8.16 Mycosis fungoides/Sézary syndrome.

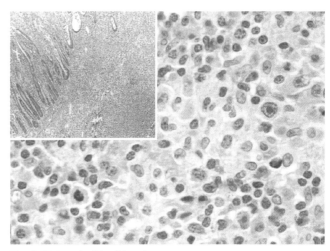

Fig. 8.17 Intestinal T cell lymphoma.

Enteropathy-type T cell lymphoma (Fig. 8.17)

Small intestinal lymphomas have long been recognized as a complication of celiac disease. They were first thought to be a heterogeneous group of tumors but later studies suggested a histiocytic origin. In the early 1980s it became clear that they were T cell lymphomas of widely varying morphology. This neoplasm is often associated with small bowel ulceration. It was formerly known as intestinal T cell lymphoma in the REAL classification. The typical histologic features of celiac disease, although often present, may be absent because of the phenomenon of "latency" recently recognized in celiac patients. In keeping with this, some patients have a history of documented celiac disease while others present with the lymphoma. The neoplastic cells express pan-T cell markers and, in most cases, the CD103 integrin molecule found on normal intestinal T lymphocytes. In most cases a proportion of the tumor cells express CD30 so care should be taken not to confuse this lesion with anaplastic large cell lymphoma. The clinical outlook is poor because the neoplasm is often multifocal.

Angioimmunoblastic T cell lymphoma

Angioimmunoblastic T cell lymphoma (Fig. 8.18) was initially thought of as an abnormal immune reaction, but is now considered as a category of peripheral T cell lymphoma in which the neoplastic cells are mixed with and obscured by a complex histologic picture including proliferating vessels, epithelioid histiocytes, plasma cells, eosinophils and hyperplastic clusters of follicular dendritic cells. The neoplastic cells are of variable morphology and include atypical "clear" cells with round nuclei and abundant pale cytoplasm. The cells carry T cell markers and are usually CD4 and CD10 positive. Patients often have systemic symptoms such as

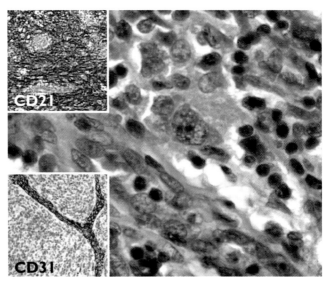

Fig. 8.18 Angioimmunoblastic T cell lymphoma.

weight loss, fever, skin rash and a polyclonal hypergammaglobulinemia. The disease is moderately aggressive and a high grade lymphoma (usually of T but occasionally of B cell type) may emerge.

Extranodal NK/T cell lymphoma nasal type

This is an extranodal lymphoma involving the nasopharynx, upper airways and soft tissues (Fig. 8.19). It was formerly called angiocentric T cell lymphoma in the REAL classification. There is a tendency to invade the walls of blood vessels, accompanied in many cases by blockage of vessels by lymphoma cells, often associated with ischemic necrosis of normal and neoplastic tissue. Virtually all cases contain EB virus, which is believed to be an important factor in the generation

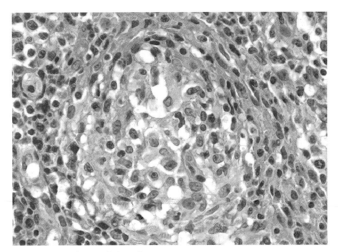

Fig. 8.19 Angiocentric lymphoma.

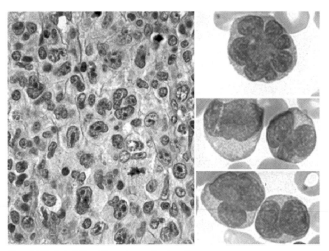

Fig. 8.20 Adult T cell lymphoma/leukemia.

of the necrosis. The origin of the neoplastic cells is unclear: T cell antigens such as CD2 and cytotoxic granule associated molecules are usually present although surface CD3 is absent in many cases. CD56, a molecule associated with NK cells, is typically expressed. The disease is rare in the USA and Europe but is much more common in Asia and Central and South America. The distinction from endemic neoplasms of large granular lymphocytes is not always clear. The disease may be curable if localized but disseminated cases have a poor prognosis.

Adult T cell leukemia/lymphoma (Fig. 8.20)

In the 1970s, an unusual T cell neoplasm was reported in South Western Japan which was subsequently shown to be confined to patients infected with the human T cell lymphoma virus type 1 (HTLV-1) retrovirus. Identical cases were then found in other areas of HTLV-1 infection, notably the Caribbean. The lymph node is diffusely replaced by neoplastic T cells, which vary widely in cell size and shape, and neoplastic cells may also be seen in the peripheral blood. Patients often have aggressive disease, associated with lytic bone lesions, and hypercalcemia, but the course is very variable and indolent or smoldering cases are seen.

Anaplastic large cell lymphoma

Anaplastic large cell lymphoma (Fig. 8.21) was first recognized as a neoplasm that was positive for the Ki-1 or CD30 antigen, an activation-associated antigen also found on Reed–Sternberg cells. The neoplastic cells can be larger than in any other type of lymphoma, and cases may be misdiagnosed as malignant histiocytosis or even anaplastic carcinoma. Distinction from Hodgkin lymphoma can also on occasion be difficult. Typically,

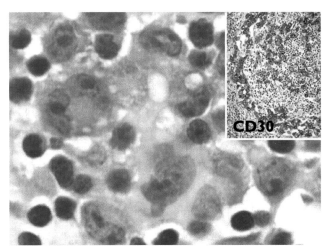

Fig. 8.21 Anaplastic large cell lymphoma.

the tumor grows in a cohesive pattern, tending to invade lymphoid sinuses, and may spread to soft tissue, bone and skin. The neoplasm may be negative for cell lineage markers, but if such antigens are present, they commonly indicate a T cell origin. In many cases there is a translocation between chromosome 2 and 5 causing fusion of the *ALK* gene with the nucleophosmin gene. There are also a number of other variant translocations in which *ALK* partners other genes. Patients can be of all ages and at least 50% of cases are seen in children or young adults. The clinical pattern is variable, some cases showing widespread involvement of lymph nodes and other sites and other cases tending to be confined to skin. The latter form of the disease which is *ALK* negative is indolent but difficult to cure, whereas the systemic type may respond to aggressive treatment.

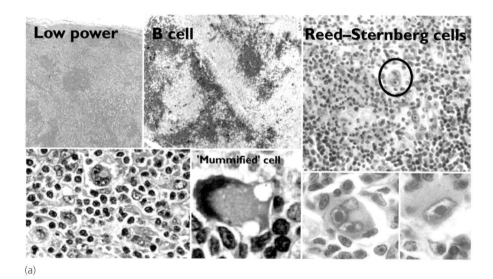

(a)

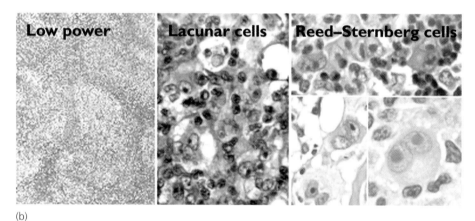

(b)

Fig. 8.22 (a) Hodgkin lymphoma, nodular sclerosis. (b) Hodgkin lymphoma, mixed cellularity.

Hodgkin lymphoma

Classic subtypes

In classical Hodgkin lymphoma, scattered binucleate or multinucleate Reed–Sternberg cells and mononuclear Hodgkin cells are seen, associated with a reactive cellular infiltrate of lymphoid cells, eosinophils and other inflammatory cells (Fig. 8.22a). The nodular sclerosis subtype is characterized by prominent fibrotic bands running through the diseased tissue, a thickened lymph node capsule and "lacunar" cells, a peculiar variant of the Reed–Sternberg cell. These features are absent in mixed cellularity Hodgkin lymphoma, in which the heterogeneous cellular infiltrate is the cardinal feature.

When this infiltrate is sparse and Reed–Sternberg cells numerous and often bizarre, the disease falls into the lymphocyte depletion category, while the reverse pattern is seen in the lymphocyte rich category. The lymphocyte depletion subtype is rare and can be difficult to distinguish from anaplastic large cell lymphoma.

In mixed cellularity Hodgkin lymphoma the node is uniformly replaced by a mixed infiltrate of abnormal and reactive cells (Fig. 8.22b). The infiltrate usually has a paracortical localization, as seen when remnants of follicles are demonstrated by immunostaining for B cell antigens. When this pattern is marked, a diagnosis is sometimes made of "interfollicular" Hodgkin lymphoma. Apoptotic or "mummified" neoplastic cells are commonly found.

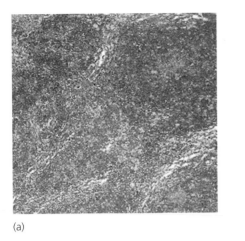 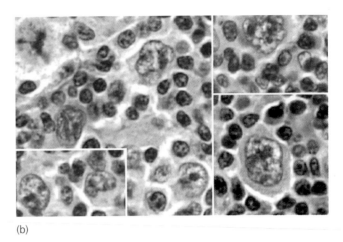

(a)   (b)

Fig. 8.23 Hodgkin lymphoma, lymphocyte predominance. (a) Low power. (b) High power.

Nodular lymphocyte predominant

Nodular lymphocyte predominant Hodgkin lymphoma (Fig. 8.23) shares with the classic subtypes of Hodgkin lymphoma a histologic picture in which scattered neoplastic cells are seen against the background of a varied reactive cellular infiltrate both within and outside of the nodules. However, most of the neoplastic cells, known as "L & H" (lymphocytic and histiocytic) or "popcorn" cells, lie within large nodular areas made up of small lymphoid cells.

References

1 Harris NL, Jaffe ES, Stein H, *et al.* A Revised European American classification of lymphoid neoplasms: A proposal from the international lymphoma study group. *Blood* 1994; **84**: 1361–92.

2 Jaffe ES, Harris NL, Stein H, *et al.* (eds). *Pathology and Genetics of Tumours of Haematopoietic and Lymphoid Tissues.* Lyon: IARC Press, 2001.

Chapter 8.2 Acute lymphoblastic leukemia and lymphoblastic lymphoma

These neoplasms may be of B (mainly the so-called pre-B) or T cell type. There has been much discussion and argument about the relationship between acute lymphoblastic leukemia (ALL) and lymphoblastic lymphoma although most of it is of little assistance when examining trephines. Most cases that present with bone marrow involvement, whether or not there is tissue infiltration, are of B cell type. The T cell lymphoblastics are rarer (less than 20% of all lymphoblastic lymphomas in most series) but give rise to the well-described clinical syndrome of mediastinal tumors without an obvious leukemic phase. Lymphoblastic lesions are aggressive and are rapidly fatal if untreated. With current treatment they are potentially curable, especially in the younger age group with ALL (both B and T).

Histopathology of the bone marrow

B and T cell cases have identical morphologic features. The neoplastic lymphoblasts are slightly larger than lymphocytes and have round or convoluted nuclei, fine chromatin often with a smudged appearance, inconspicuous nucleoli and scant, faintly basophilic cytoplasm. Mitotic figures are numerous (Fig. 8.24). The marrow is packed with little of the hematopoietic tissue or fat remaining although occasionally a more patchy infiltration is evident (Fig. 8.25). Areas of necrosis (often a sinister sign in a marrow) may be present. The distinction between B and T cell cases can only be made immunocytochemically (Fig. 8.26).

An important practical note is that B lymphoblasts have a precursor phenotype being CD79a positive with mature B markers such as CD20 either being absent or weak and patchily expressed (Fig. 8.26). Surprisingly (for pathologists) T cell ALL is also frequently positive for CD79a[1] but the presence of T cell markers such as CD3 and CD7 and the frequent coexpression (or absence) of CD4 and CD8 reveal its true nature (Fig. 8.26). CD10 is also present on a large number of T cell ALLs (Fig. 8.26) and may be absent on cases of B cell ALL (Fig. 8.27).

Immunophenotype B cell: TdT+, CD10+/–, CD19+ CD20–/+, CD22–, CD79a+, Sig–
Immunophenotype T cell: TdT+, CD3+, CD7+, CD10–/+ CD2 & 5 variable, CD4+/–, CD8+/– CD79a–/+

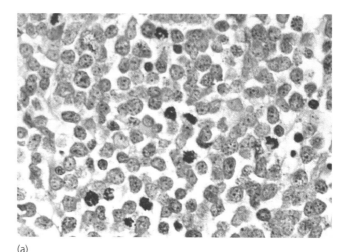

(a)

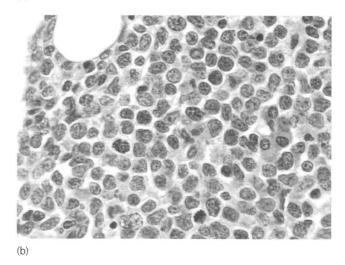

(b)

Fig. 8.24 Cytology of lymphoblastic lymphoma. (a) Giemsa. (b) H&E.

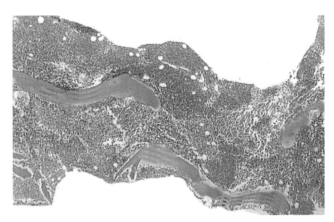

Fig. 8.25 Hypercellular marrow in lymphoblastic lymphoma. H&E.

B cell ALL

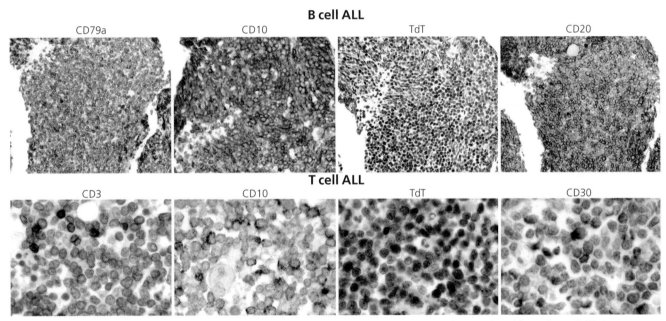

Fig. 8.26 Top row: B cell acute lymphoblastic leukemia (ALL) stained for CD79a, CD10 and terminal deoxynucleotidyl transferase (TdT). Some cases are also CD20 positive although usually rather weakly and patchily. Bottom row: T cell ALL stained for CD3, CD10 and TdT. A number of other antigens may be present such as coexpression of CD4 and CD8 (not shown) or CD30.

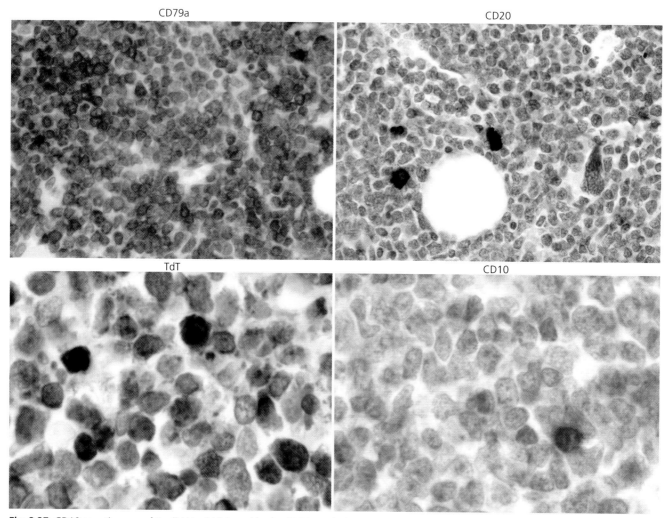

Fig. 8.27 CD10 negative case of B cell ALL which is positive for CD79a and TdT but negative for CD20. All T cell markers were absent.

Diagnostic problems

1 *Sparse infiltrate.* Occasionally, the infiltrate is sparse with blast cells outnumbered by normal marrow cells so that it is easy for the histopathologist to overlook them. This may occur at diagnosis as well as at early relapse and is relatively easily recognized by immunostaining for B or T cell antigens (Fig. 8.28) and TdT.

2 *Distinction from chronic lymphoblastic leukemia (CLL).* The small size of the lymphoblasts and the packed nature of the marrow can produce a picture in an adult that is surprisingly easy to confuse with CLL, although this does not seem to have been admitted in print. It can be avoided by checking for a high mitotic rate in ALL which will be confirmed by abundant positively stained nuclei for proliferation markers such as Ki67 (Fig. 8.29).

3 *Distinction from acute myeloid leukemia (AML).* Histologically AML looks like ALL. The key to distinguishing these two important conditions is careful immunophenotyping as detailed in this chapter for ALL and Chapter 7 for AML. It must be emphasized that these very primitive tumors resolutely refuse to obey any rules given them and immunophenotypic exceptions are increasingly going to be found (Fig. 8.30).

4 *Detection of early disease and relapse.* Sometimes patients, especially children, have a prodromal illness where leukemia is suspected but not diagnosed until sometime later (Fig. 8.31). Careful examination of the marrow from these early occurrences will often highlight foci of what in retrospect is ALL. It must be said, however, that it would take a brave pathologist to make a firm diagnosis on a case such as this.

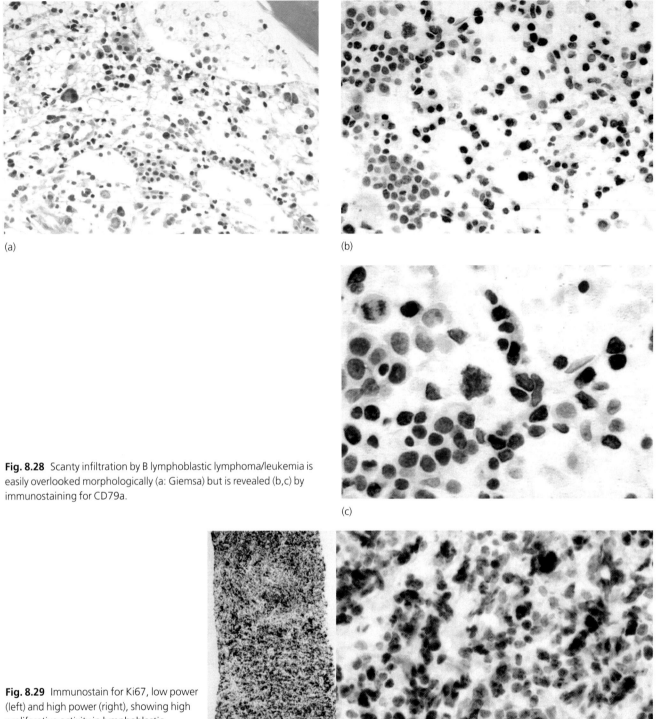

(a)

(b)

(c)

Fig. 8.28 Scanty infiltration by B lymphoblastic lymphoma/leukemia is easily overlooked morphologically (a: Giemsa) but is revealed (b,c) by immunostaining for CD79a.

Fig. 8.29 Immunostain for Ki67, low power (left) and high power (right), showing high proliferative activity in lymphoblastic lymphoma.

CD79a

TdT

c-kit (CD117)

myeloperoxidase

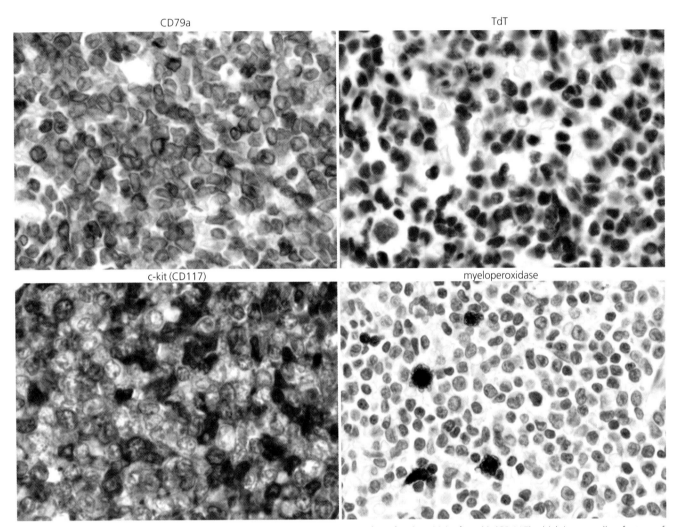

Fig. 8.30 Case of B cell ALL with a typical cytology and immunophenotype apart from focal positivity for c-kit (CD117) which is generally a feature of AML. This case is myeloperoxidase negative.

Original presentation

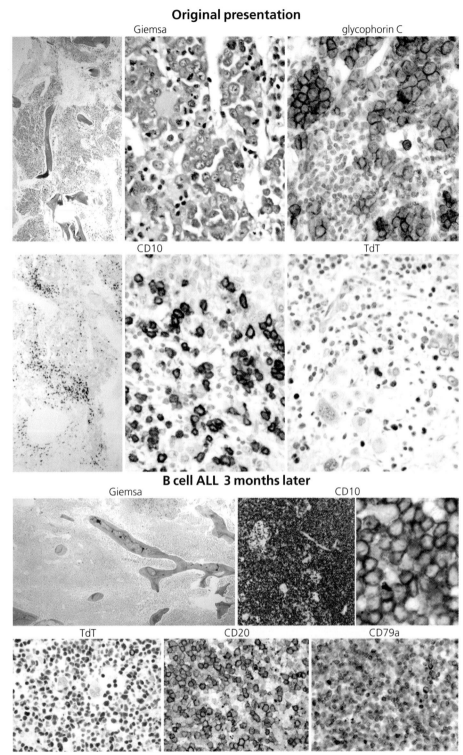

Fig. 8.31 A 4-year-old girl presented with pancytopenia and a few blasts in the peripheral blood. The marrow is hyperplastic but the blasts are predominantly erythroid (glycophorin C) although careful inspection showed a few focal areas of CD10 positivity within which there were a few TdT positive cells. A cautious descriptive report of an abnormal marrow was issued but within 3 months frank B cell ALL, as shown below, emerged.

Caution is also urged when examining marrows after treatment, especially in children. Regenerative change in the marrow often leads to a number of precursor B cells (often referred to as hematagones) that can have an identical phenotype to ALL (i.e. CD10+, TdT+ and CD79a+). These precursor cells can occasionally be seen in otherwise normal or unrelated marrows. There is a good discussion of this diagnostic problem in the WHO book to which the interested reader is referred.[2]

Key points

- Aggressive but potentially curable disease.
- Small blast cells with high mitotic rate.
- Packed marrow (often virtually a total replacement).
- May resemble CLL at low power.

References

1 Pilozzi E, Pulford KAF, Jones M, *et al.* Co-expression of CD79a (JCB117) and CD3 by lymphoblastic lymphoma. *J Pathol* 1998; **182**: 140–3.

2 Jaffe ES, Harris NL, Stein H, *et al.* (eds). *Pathology and Genetics of Tumours of Haematopoietic and Lymphoid Tissues*: Lyon: IARC Press, 2001.

Chapter 8.3 Chronic lymphocytic leukemia

The separation of small lymphocytic lymphoma (SLL) and chronic lymphocytic leukemia (CLL) is arbitrary and is based on the tissue involved (i.e. SLL is restricted to cases with the tissue morphology and immunophenotype of CLL but which is non-leukemic). Some patients may have disease restricted to one site although the majority will show evidence of marrow involvement. It should be remembered that the neoplastic cell is morphologically and immunophenotypically identical in all of these settings. It is for this reason that major lymphoma classifications such as the Revised European and American Lymphoma (REAL) or Kiel use the term CLL for all aspects of this disease. The neoplastic cell is usually (99%) a B cell. The rare T cell variant is difficult to recognize on cell morphology alone.

Clinical features

This is the most frequent leukemia in Europe and North America. It is more common in men and the median age at diagnosis is 60 years. Patients may present with tiredness, breathlessness, enlarged lymph nodes and in the later stages with bleeding problems and infections. Mild to moderate hepatosplenomegaly may be present. In T cell CLL, skin involvement may occur. In prolymphocytic leukemia (PLL), splenomegaly is often marked but lymphadenopathy is uncommon.

Histopathology of the bone marrow

Marrow involved by CLL is generally hypercellular. Residual marrow elements are usually present unless the disease is advanced in which case the marrow spaces are packed with neoplastic cells. Several patterns of involvement have been described (i.e. interstitial, nodular, mixed (interstitial and nodular) and diffuse). These patterns recognize marrow involvement at different stages of disease progression. The most frequent pattern at presentation is mixed. The marrow contains aggregates of the neoplastic cells and also has a back-

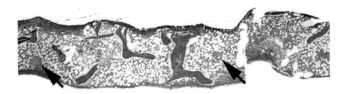

(a)

(b)

Fig. 8.32 Early presentation of chronic lymphocytic leukemia (CLL) with small, centrally located nodules (arrows).
(a) Low power. (b) Medium power.

ground infiltrate throughout the marrow intimately admixed with the hematopoietic tissue. The aggregates usually have a central distribution within the marrow space (Fig. 8.32) although as they increase in size they will eventually expand into contact with the endosteum (Fig. 8.33).

The neoplastic cell is a small lymphocyte with a round nucleus, clumped chromatin and inconspicuous nucleolus (Fig. 8.34). It has a characteristic immunophenotype being positive for CD20, CD23 and CD5 (Fig. 8.35) but negative for CD3 (thus not a T cell tumor) and cyclin D1 (distinguishing it from mantle cell lymphoma) (Fig. 8.36).

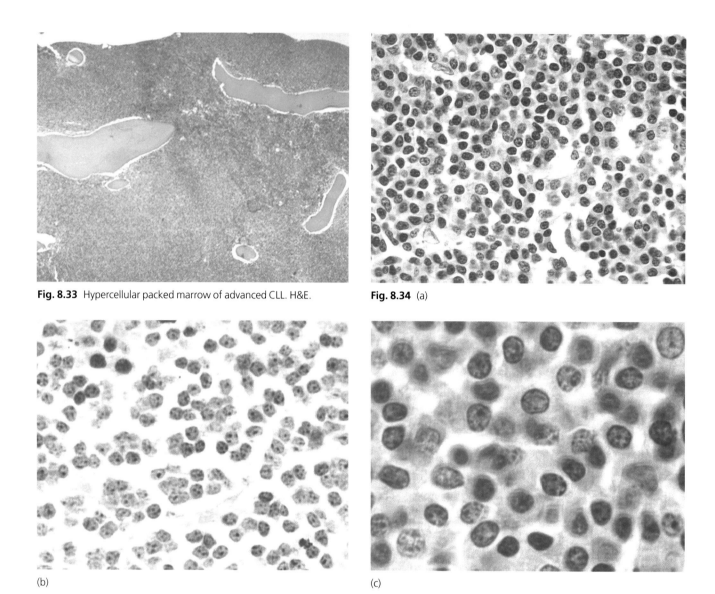

Fig. 8.33 Hypercellular packed marrow of advanced CLL. H&E.

Fig. 8.34 (a)

(b)

(c)

Fig. 8.34 Cytologic appearances of CLL in bone marrow sections. (a–c) Giemsa.

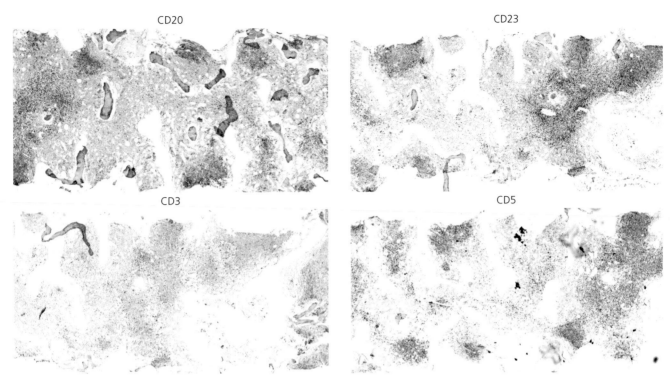

Fig. 8.35 Immunophenotype of CLL shows typically positivity for CD20, CD23 and CD5 but negativity for CD3.

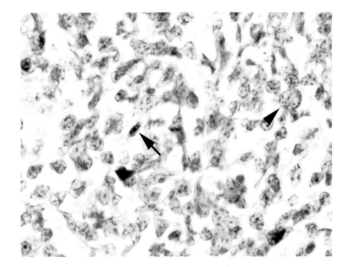

Fig. 8.36 CLL is negative for cyclin D1 distinguishing it from mantle cell lymphoma. Note the positive nuclei in endothelial cells (arrow) and macrophages (arrowhead) which provide an inbuilt positive control.

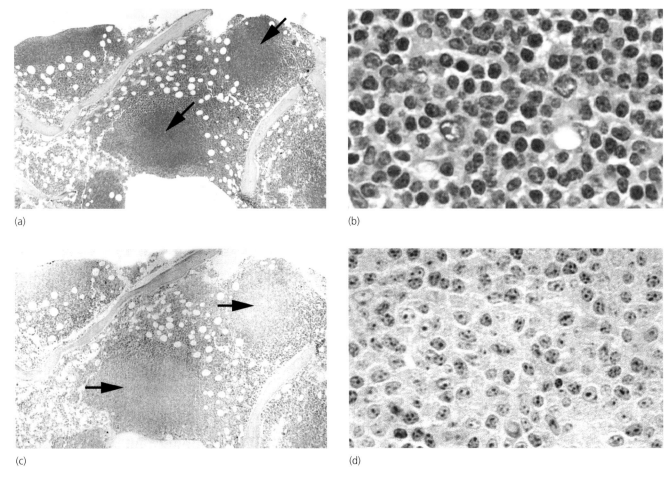

(a)

(b)

(c)

(d)

Fig. 8.37 Proliferation centers (arrows) in CLL. (a,b) H&E. (c,d) Giemsa.

The proliferation centers, containing larger prolymphocytes and paraimmunoblasts that are an obvious part of nodal disease, are occasionally seen in the bone marrow (Fig. 8.37).

One distinguishing feature of T cell CLL (or PLL, as most cases are prolymphocytic rather than lymphocytic) is that it does not form proliferation centers. In patients with peripheral destruction of platelets in enlarged spleens it is possible to see a reactive hyperplasia of the megakaryocytic series in the bone marrow. Richter syndrome, the transformation of CLL to a large cell lymphoma usually still demonstrably B cell, occurs in a small proportion of cases (Fig. 8.38).

Variations such as PLL are more reliably identified on smears. These patients have more aggressive disease and respond less well to the treatment regimens used for CLL. Prolymphocytes, which must form more than half of the neoplastic cell population, have a prominent central nucleolus and more cytoplasm than CLL cells (Fig. 8.39a).

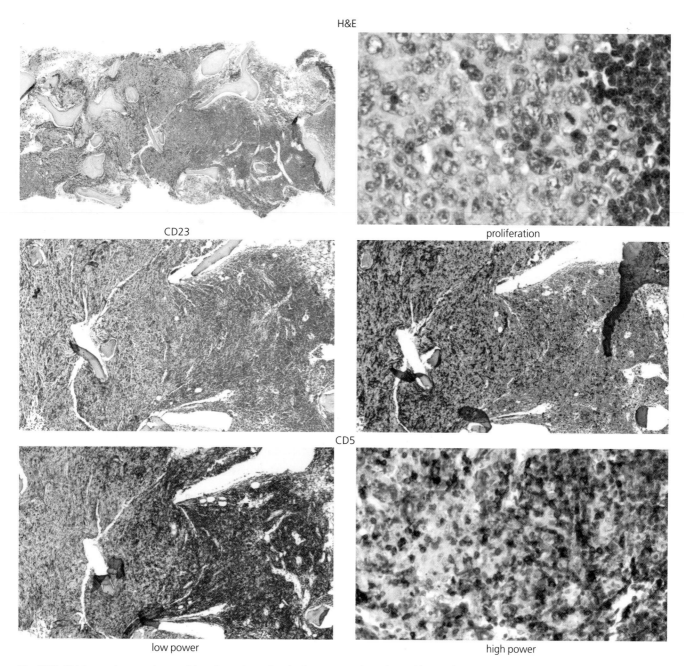

Fig. 8.38 Richter syndrome: a large cell lymphoma has arisen in the marrow of a patient with typical CLL. In all of the images the large B cell transformation (CD20 positive—not shown) is on the left and residual CLL on the right. It can be seen that the large cell lymphoma has largely lost CD5 and CD23 but has a much higher proliferation rate (Ki67) than the underlying CLL.

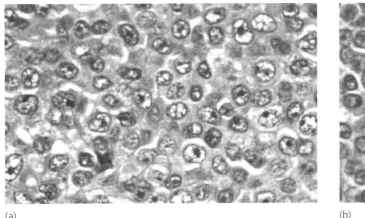

(a)

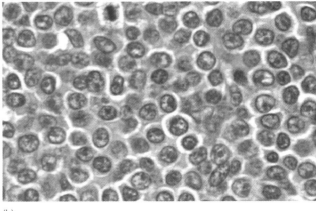

(b)

Fig. 8.39a The appearances of prolymphocytic leukemia (PLL) cells in bone marrow trephine sections from two separate cases.

Many cases of CLL show a degree of plasmacytic differentiation yet have the same immunophenotype as typical CLL. There does not appear to be any difference in the clinical behavior of these cases from typical CLL. These cases were separately classified in the Kiel scheme as lymphoplasmacytoid lymphoma but are considered to be the same entity in both the REAL and WHO classifications. They differ from lymphoplasmacytic lymphoma (Waldenström macroglobulinemia) both morphologically and immunophenotypically.

Diagnostic problems

Distinction between reactive lymphoid nodules and CLL

In CLL the number of nodules is usually more than three in a trephine of >1 cm in length, although confirmation of clonality may be needed to confirm the diagnosis. Other histologic features that may be helpful have been discussed previously (see Chapter 2).

Is it possible to distinguish between CLL and small cell lymphocytic lymphoma on marrow histology?

There are no definite features that allow a reliable distinction to be made.

Distinguishing T cell from B cell PLL

The WHO book says this is difficult to perform by bone marrow histology alone but for lesser mortals the word impossible (or

> *Immunophenotype:* CD19+, CD20+, CD79a+, CD5+, CD23+, CD43+, cyclin D1−

maybe inadvisable) might be more accurate. In fact a simple immunophenotypic study will sort them out (Fig. 8.39b).

Distinguishing between cytopenias that are immune based and those resulting from loss of hematopoietic tissue

Some patients with CLL develop cytopenias. In those cases where this is results from loss of hematopoietic tissue, the marrow will show replacement of the normal blood-forming cell lines by malignant cells. In those cases where the cytopenias are immune-based and the blood cells are being destroyed, a hyperplastic picture may be seen with the affected cell lines displaying increased numbers of their more immature members in an attempt to replace the cells destroyed peripherally.

Distinguishing between CLL and small cell acute leukemias

On histology alone it is surprisingly easy to misdiagnose ALL as CLL especially in an adult where the former is unexpected. Full knowledge of the clinical picture and close inspection of the cell morphology will prevent such a mistake (although it is unlikely one would get such a howler past a competent hematologist!). Mitotic figures will be obvious in acute leukemia and virtually absent in CLL. The immunophenotypes are also entirely different.

Giemsa   CD5

CD3   CD2

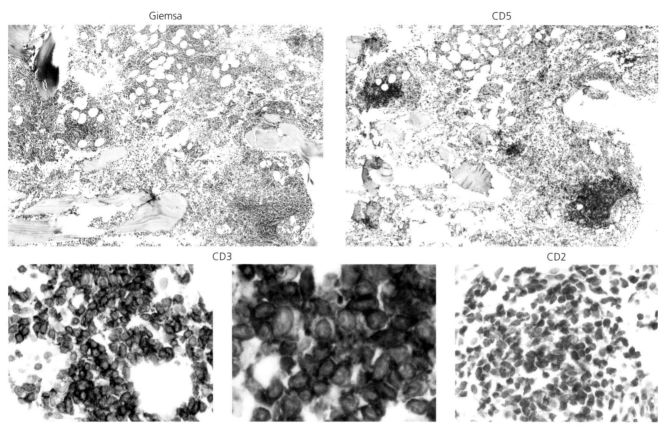

Fig. 8.39b T cell PLL showing a characteristic CLL-like nodular infiltration of the marrow with the prolymphocytes being positive for CD5, CD3 (shown at high power as well) and CD2.

Key points

- This is a low-grade, indolent lymphoma/leukemia although it is currently incurable.
- Nearly all cases are B cell.
- The marrow is hypercellular and usually has a nodular pattern.
- The nodules have a central, intertrabecular distribution.
- CLL variants are difficult to identify on marrow histology.

Chapter 8.4 Lymphoplasmacytic lymphoma

(including Waldenström macroglobulinemia)

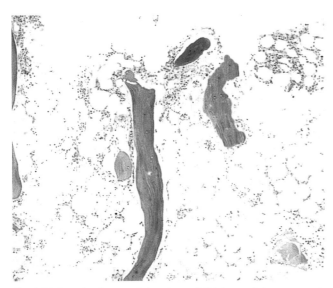

Fig. 8.41 Lymphoplasmacytic lymphoma (LPL): hypocellular marrow at presentation. Giemsa.

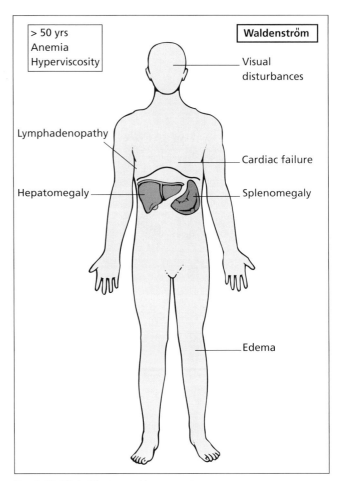

> 50 yrs
Anemia
Hyperviscosity

Waldenström

Visual disturbances

Lymphadenopathy

Cardiac failure

Hepatomegaly

Splenomegaly

Edema

Fig. 8.40 Clinical features of immunocytoma.

This low-grade B cell malignancy shows a particular tendency towards plasma cell differentiation. Although commonly involving lymph nodes it typically presents in the bone marrow where it is often associated with the clinical syndrome of Waldenström macroglobulinemia. This is characterized by an immunoglobulin M (IgM) paraprotein in the serum. These patients usually present with increasing tiredness. The large IgM protein molecules increase the blood's viscosity, producing visual disturbances and cardiac failure. There is often lymphadenopathy and hepatosplenomegaly (Fig. 8.40). Occasionally, other types of lymphoma, especially chronic lymphocytic leukemia (CLL), may be associated with Waldenström macroglobulinemia.[1]

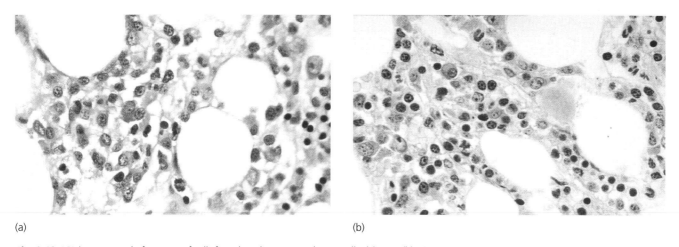

(a)   (b)

Fig. 8.42 LPL is composed of a range of cells from lymphocytes to plasma cells. (a) H&E. (b) Giemsa.

Histopathology of the bone marrow

At presentation the marrow is often hypocellular (Fig. 8.41) but becomes increasingly infiltrated as the disease progresses. The normal hematopoietic tissue is replaced by neoplastic B cells showing a range of differentiation between lymphocytes and plasma cells (Fig. 8.42) which appropriate immunostains will highlight dramatically. In fact the differential expression of a plasma cell marker such as VS38 (p63) or CD138 can be very effective in differentiating immunocytoma from other B cell lymphomas (with little positivity) and myeloma (where all neoplastic cells are positive) (Fig. 8.43).

IgM and light chain restriction can be demonstrated immunohistochemically in the neoplastic cells, particularly in the more plasmacytic forms (Fig. 8.44). Some of the plasmacytoid cells and plasma cells contain perinuclear accumulations of IgM which indent the nucleus and appear to be intranuclear (Dutcher bodies) (Fig. 8.45).

Early involvement is frequently patchy, sometimes resembling CLL with centrally located nodules and at other times follicular lymphoma with paratrabecular aggregations. There is also a sparse diffuse infiltrate spreading through the rest of the marrow easily seen with immunocytochemical assistance (Fig. 8.46). As the disease progresses this enlarges to fill the entire marrow.

Two additional features may be seen in association with the neoplastic cell infiltrate:
1 Mast cells are often numerous. They are best seen in a Giemsa-stained section as this reveals the metachromatic properties of the cell's granules. Although these cells are increased in a number of other lymphoproliferative conditions that affect the bone marrow, they are particularly numerous in Waldenström macroglobulinemia (Fig. 8.47).
2 Within the interstitium there is deposition of an amorphous, eosinophilic, periodic acid–Schiff (PAS) positive substance, probably IgM (Fig. 8.48).

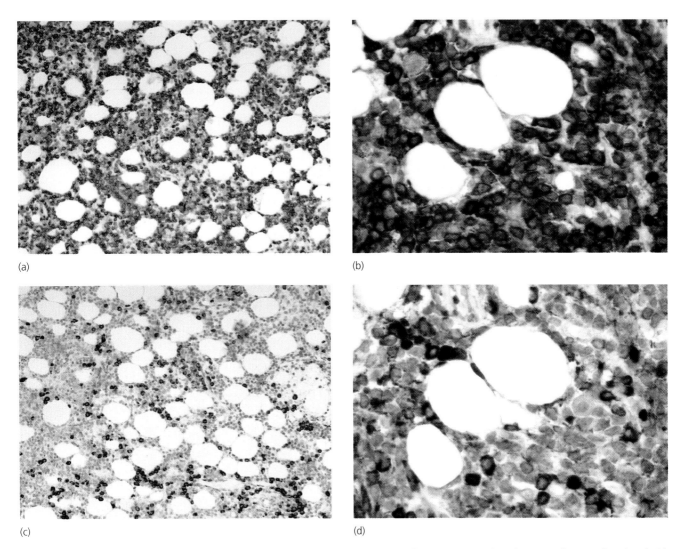

(a)

(b)

(c)

(d)

Fig. 8.43 LPL is a B cell proliferation (a,b: CD79) which shows a characteristic expression of the antigen p63 (VS38), ranging from weak on lymphoid to strong on plasma cells. (c,d) Immunostain for p63 (VS38).

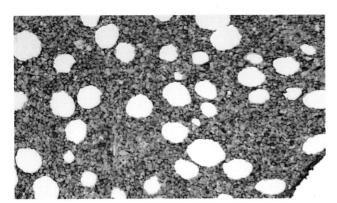

Fig. 8.44 Kappa light chain restriction in LPL.

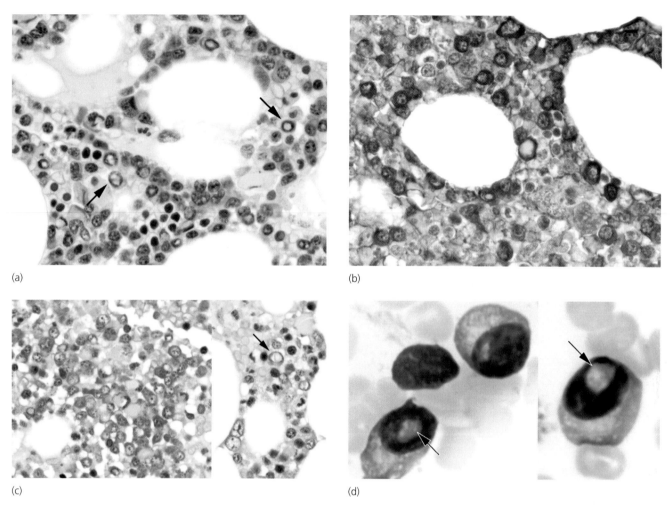

Fig. 8.45 Dutcher bodies (arrows) in LPL seen on both histology and smear cytology. Light chain staining demonstrates their clonality. (a) H&E, (b) lambda, (c) Giemsa, (d) smear.

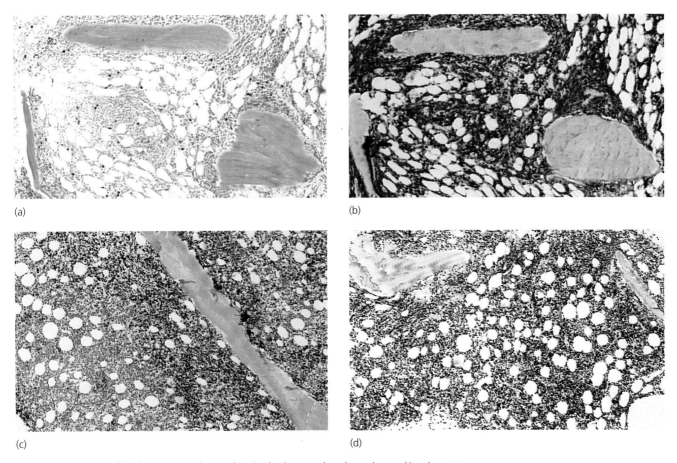

(a)

(b)

(c)

(d)

Fig. 8.46 Infiltration of the bone marrow by LPL showing both paratrabecular and central involvement.
(a) Giemsa. (b) CD79a (B cell). (c,d) VS38 (p63).

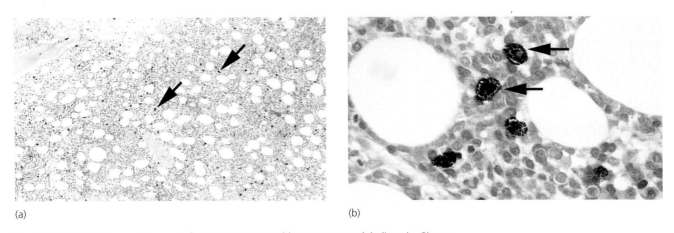

(a)

(b)

Fig. 8.47 Mast cells (arrows) in a case of LPL giving rise to Waldenström macroglobulinemia. Giemsa.

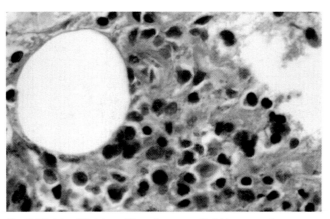

Fig. 8.48 Interstitial deposition of presumed IgM in a case of Waldenström macroglobulinemia. Periodic acid–Schiff (PAS).

Immunophenotype: positive for surface and cytoplasmic Ig (usually IgM), CD19, CD20, CD22, CD79a. They typically lack CD5 and CD10.* The strong cytoplasmic Ig staining and lack of CD5 help distinguish it from B cell chronic lymphocytic leukemia (B-CLL).

* A recent publication suggests that a small number of cases of lymphoplasmacytic lymphoma may express CD5 or CD10,[2] although this will need confirming by other studies.

Key points

- The neoplastic cells have features of both small lymphocytes and plasma cells.
- The neoplastic cells produce cytoplasmic Ig (usually IgM) and lack CD5.
- Mast cells are often very prominent.

References

1 Lin P, Hao S, Handy BC, *et al.* Lymphoid neoplasms associated with IgM paraprotein: a study of 382 patients. *Am J Clin Pathol* 2005; **123**: 200–5.

2 Konoplev S, Medeiros LJ, Bueso-Ramos CE, *et al.* Immunophenotypic profile of lymphoplasmacytic lymphoma/Waldenström macroglobulinemia. *Am J Clin Pathol* 2005; **124**: 414–20.

Chapter 8.5 Mantle cell lymphoma

This was known as centrocytic lymphoma by the Kiel group who originally described it. Prior to this it had been regarded by many as a lymphoma showing differentiation intermediate between CLL and follicular lymphoma. The neoplastic cells are now believed to originate from the mantle zone and not from the germinal centre. Most cases have a t(11;14) translocation which appears to activate cyclin D1 (this is a cell cycle protein not usually expressed in lymphoid cells). Cyclin D1 is also raised in cases without this translocation, indicating that other mechanisms may also be involved.

It generally occurs in adults over 50 years, often male, and is usually widespread at diagnosis. It involves lymph nodes, spleen, Waldeyer ring, bone marrow and the gastrointestinal tract (lymphomatous polyposis). It has a more aggressive course than other low grade lymphomas and is generally incurable (Fig. 8.49).

It does not seem to transform to large cell lymphoma but a small to medium-sized blast cell variant may occur which has an even worse prognosis.

Histopathology of the bone marrow

The marrow infiltrate consists of a uniform population of small to medium lymphoid cells with cleaved or angular nuclei, dispersed chromatin, inconspicuous nucleoli and scanty cytoplasm (Fig. 8.50).

Unlike follicular lymphoma virtually no larger cells (i.e. centroblasts) are present. Marrow involvement may be both paratrabecular and diffuse (Fig. 8.51).

A small number of cases (blastoid variant) have cells with slightly larger nuclei, more dispersed chromatin and a higher proliferation index and to some extent resemble lymphoblasts (Fig. 8.52).

> *Immunophenotype:* positive for surface IgM, CD19, 20, 22, 79a, CD5, CD43, bcl2 and cyclin D1 and negative for CD23, CD10 and bcl6

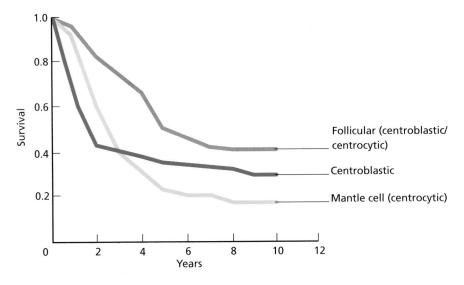

Follicular (centroblastic/ centrocytic)

Centroblastic

Mantle cell (centrocytic)

Fig. 8.49 Mantle cell lymphoma survival curve.

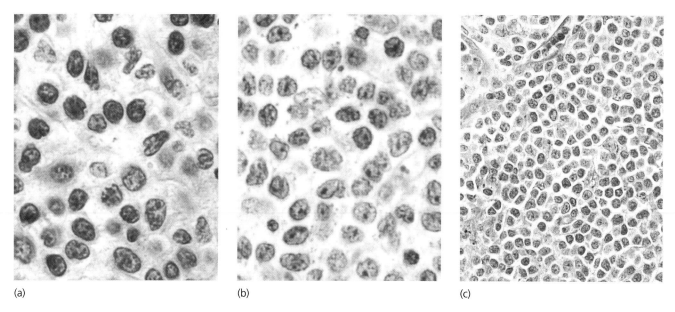

(a)

(b)

(c)

Fig. 8.50 Cytologic appearances of mantle cell lymphoma. (a) H&E. (b) Giemsa. Note the characteristic gray low-power appearance on Giemsa staining (c).

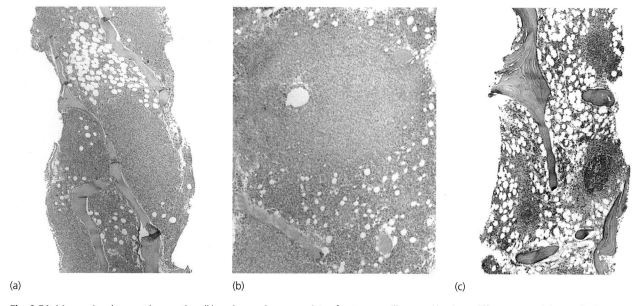

(a)

(b)

(c)

Fig. 8.51 Marrow involvement by mantle cell lymphoma shows a variety of patterns as illustrated by three different cases. (a) H&E. (b,c) Giemsa.

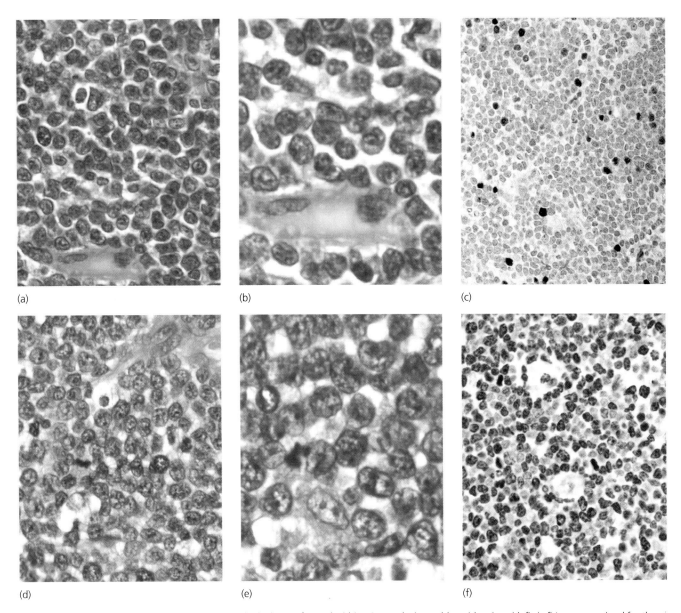

(a) (b) (c)

(d) (e) (f)

Fig. 8.52 Typical case of mantle cell lymphoma (a–c) which transformed within 12 months into a blastoid variant (d–f). (c,f) Immunostained for the proliferation associated antigen Ki67.

Diagnostic problems

Distinguishing CLL, follicular lymphoma and MCL is usually achieved in nodal tissue by an examination of the architecture and cell morphology. This is more difficult on a trephine biopsy. Immunohistochemistry for CD5, CD23 and cyclin D1 is essential for distinguishing these tumours (Table 8.4) (Fig. 8.53).

Nuclear positivity for cyclin D1 has become particularly useful to the histologist but two points need currently to be borne in mind. First, new antibodies combined with advances in antigen retrieval have greatly augmented the detection of this hitherto difficult to detect antigen. This means that one needs to distinguish background endothelial and macrophage nuclei which are normally positive from lymphoma cells. Second, the controversy as to whether or not some cases of mantle cell lymphoma can be cyclin D1 negative may have been resolved. Recent molecular studies have shown that a few cases with the genetic fingerprint of mantle cell lymphoma may lack the t(11;14) and express cyclin D2 or D3 while being negative for cyclin D1.[1]

Table 8.4 Differential diagnosis of small B cell lymphoma.

	CLL	Follicular lymphoma	MCL
CD5	+	−	+
CD23	+	−/+	−
Cyclin D1	−	−	+
CD10	−	+	−

MCL, mantle cell lymphoma.

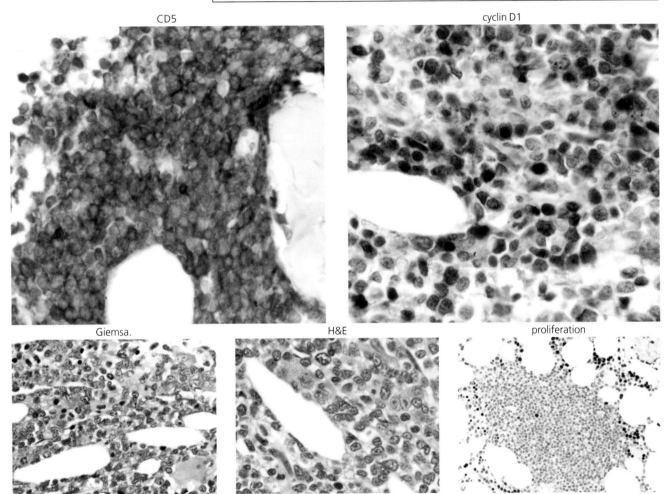

CD5   cyclin D1

Giemsa.   H&E   proliferation

Fig. 8.53 Immunophenotype of mantle cell lymphoma showing positivity for CD5 and cyclin D1. Note that typical cases have a low proliferation rate (Ki67) belying their often aggressive clinical course.

Key points

- Morphologically, the neoplastic cell may resemble a centrocyte or lymphocyte.
- MCL has a more aggressive clinical course than most other lymphomas.
- Rare blastoid variants have an even worse prognosis.
- Immunohistochemistry may be required to differentiate between CLL and follicular lymphoma.

Reference

1   Fu K, Weisenburger DD, Greiner TC, *et al.* Cyclin D1-negative mantle cell lymphoma: a clinicopathological study based on gene expression profiling. *Blood* 2005;**106** (**13**):4315–4321

Chapter 8.6 Follicular lymphoma

Follicular lymphoma is defined in the World Health Organization (WHO) classification as a neoplasm of follicle center cells that has at least a partially follicular (nodular) pattern. It is also known as centroblastic/centrocytic lymphoma in the Kiel classification. Follicular lymphoma is the most common type of non-Hodgkin lymphoma in the West and constitutes about one-third of all NHLs.

Follicular lymphoma affects adults, usually over 40 years old. It predominantly involves lymph nodes but the spleen, bone marrow (in approximately 40% of cases) and occasionally peripheral blood and extranodal sites may be involved. This lymphoma has a generally indolent although incurable clinical course. Those cases that display a greater degree of follicle formation and have fewer large cells forming the lymphoma population appear to have a better prognosis than those with a less nodular pattern and more large centroblast-like cells. Some cases may transform into a high-grade diffuse large cell lymphoma.

Histopathology of the bone marrow

These lymphomas are composed of two cell types: centrocytes (cleaved follicle center cells) and centroblasts (large non-cleaved follicle center cells). The centrocytes typically predominate (Fig. 8.54). The distribution is characteristic. The lymphoma cells are seen to lie against the trabeculae in little "drifts" which obliterate the first fat space (Fig. 8.55).

In marrows with extensive involvement these infiltrates increase in size and coalesce to fill the marrow space, gradually losing the characteristic paratrabecular pattern. The nodular pattern of growth seen in lymph nodes is rarely as convincing in the bone marrow even when the infiltrate has virtually filled the whole trephine (Fig. 8.56).

It is recognized that follicular lymphoma may undergo transformation into a large cell non-Hodgkin lymphoma (NHL). Identification of this depends on increased numbers of centroblasts which should constitute more than 50% of the lymphoma cell population. Quite frequently there will be a discordance between the bone marrow findings and the tissue diagnosis, usually when the latter is a diffuse large B cell lymphoma. This should be recorded and highlighted in the bone marrow report.

> *Immunophenotype:* surface Ig+, CD19+, bcl2+, bcl6+, CD20+, CD22+, CD79a+, CD10+/−, CD5−, CD23−/+, CD43− and CD11c−

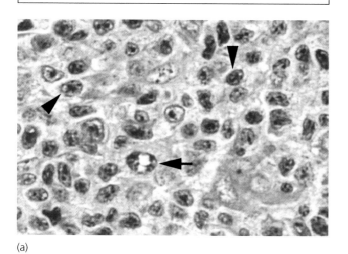

(a)

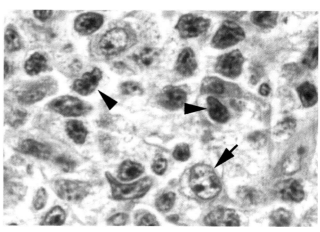

(b)

Fig. 8.54 (a,b) Centroblasts (arrow) and centrocytes (arrowheads) in a follicular lymphoma in bone marrow. Giemsa.

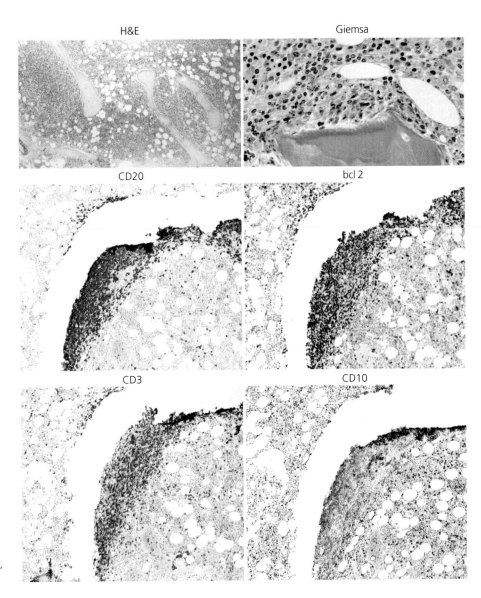

Fig. 8.55 The paratrabecular location of follicular lymphoma in bone marrow is highlighted by immunostaining for CD20, CD3, CD10 and bcl2.

Diagnostic problems

The two main difficulties are in the distinction from reactive nodules and from chronic lymphocytic leukemia (CLL). In the former, the most useful guide is the paratrabecular distribution of follicular lymphoma which, if it does occur in reactive cases, is rare.[1] Although the detection of bcl2 protein is useful in distinguishing reactive from neoplastic nodules in lymph nodes (germinal centers are bcl2 negative) it is generally not helpful in the marrow because germinal center formation is rare and both small reactive or neoplastic groups of cells may be bcl2 positive. bcl6 similarly is not helpful in this distinction.

Demonstration of light chain restriction will confirm the diagnosis but this may be difficult on fixed paraffin or resin embedded trephines.

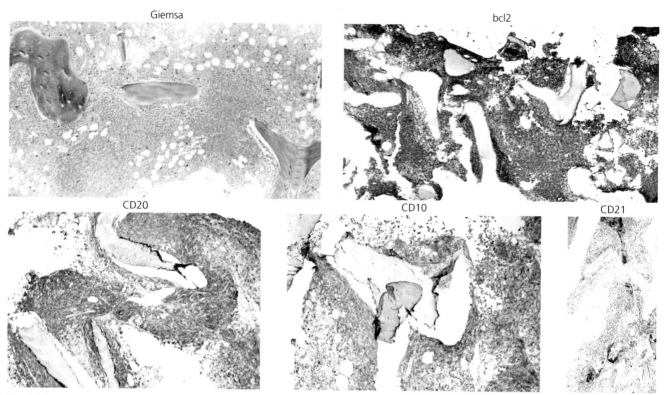

Fig. 8.56 Extensive infiltration of bone marrow by follicular lymphoma demonstrating both a nodular and diffuse pattern on Giemsa and immunostaining for bcl2, CD20 and CD10. Note that when it becomes this extensive, follicular dendritic cells can often be detected (CD21).

Immunocytochemistry is more useful in confirming the diagnosis by showing the typical paratrabecular distribution of the neoplastic B cells which may be virtually invisible to ordinary morphologic examination (Fig. 8.57). This has an additional value in the early stages of marrow involvement by highlighting the affected areas, allowing the typical centrocyte morphology of the lymphoma cells to be appreciated (Fig. 8.58).[2]

CLL usually forms round lymphoid aggregates with a central, intertrabecular distribution and is only occasionally paratrabecular. Immunophenotyping, as described in Chapter 8.3 for CLL and here for follicular lymphoma, should help make this distinction. It may be useful to comment on CD10 immunostaining in the bone marrow. Many cases of follicular lymphoma in the bone marrow are negative for CD10 and even in those cases that show positivity the amount is much less than the CD20 staining (Fig. 8.59). This should be taken into account when considering this differential diagnosis.

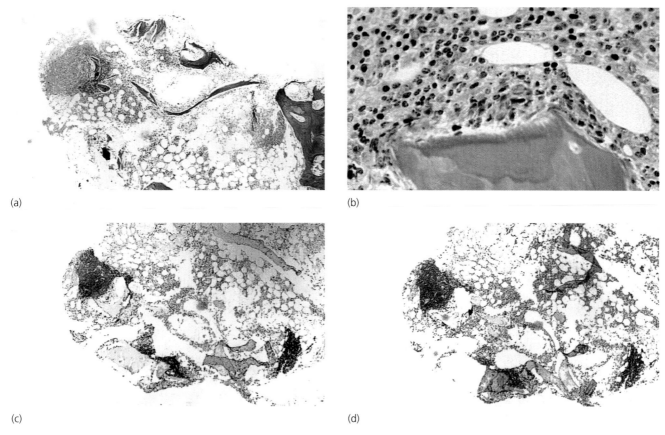

(a)

(b)

(c)

(d)

Fig. 8.57 Minimal involvement of the bone marrow by follicular lymphoma may be difficult to detect morphologically (a,b: H&E) but can be readily identified by immunostaining. (c) CD79. (d) bcl2.

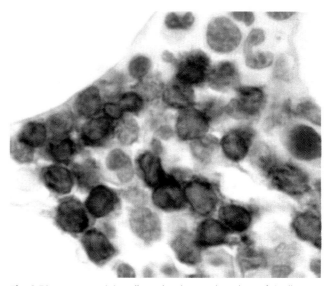

Fig. 8.58 Immunostaining allows the abnormal cytology of small deposits of follicular lymphoma to be identified. CD79.

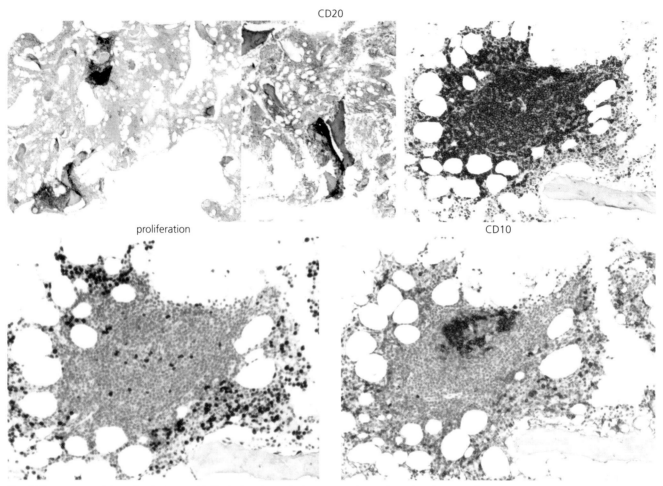

CD20

proliferation

CD10

Fig. 8.59 Immunostaining of typical case of follicular lymphoma in the marrow shows the reduced extent of CD10 staining in relation to CD20. The explanation for this is unknown at present.

The effect of rituximab treatment

A major advance in follicular (and other B cell) lymphoma therapy has come from the administration of anti-CD20 antibodies (known as rituximab) with or without chemotherapy. This gives rise to a depletion of CD20 positive cells in the marrow, even though it may look as though the follicular lymphoma is still present because of the residual accompanying T cells which are not (at least initially) eliminated (Fig. 8.60).

A population of residual B cells from which the marrow lymphocyte population recovers can be detected by staining for CD79a or PAX5. Sometimes from their distribution and number they clearly appear to represent persistent CD20 follicular lymphoma although much more clinical follow-up of these cases is needed to assess the importance of the various patterns of staining detected after rituximab treatment.

References

1 Anagnostou D. Pitfalls in the pattern of bone marrow infiltration in lymphoproliferative disorders. *Curr Diagn Pathol* 2005; **11**: 170–9.

2 Chetty R, Echezarreta G, Comley M, *et al.* Immunohistochemistry in apparently normal bone marrow trephine specimens from patients with nodal follicular lymphoma. *J Clin Pathol* 1995; **48**: 1035–8.

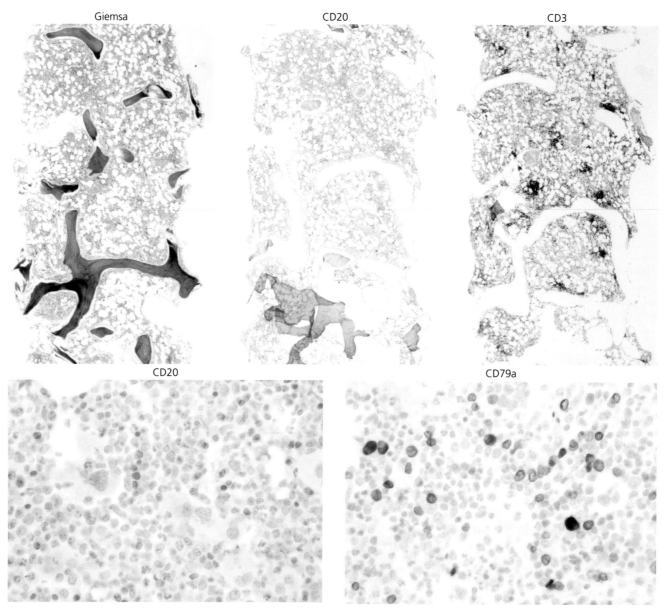

Fig. 8.60 A case of follicular lymphoma treated with rituximab some weeks before. Although the original marrow had been extensively involved, the post treatment specimen still looks as though there is considerable residual disease (Giemsa). However, immunostaining shows the residual lymphocytes are mainly T cells (CD3) with CD20+ B cells being absent. The patient's immune system recovers by using the underlying B stem cells here shown by CD79a staining (from where presumably the follicular lymphomas also often recur).

Chapter 8.7 Marginal zone B cell lymphoma (including MALT type)

The World Health Organization (WHO) classification recognizes three forms of "marginal zone B-cell lymphoma"; the extranodal type of mucosa-associated lymphoid tissue (MALT), the splenic type and the nodal type (also known as monocytoid B cell lymphoma). These are probably the same condition with different clinical features. It is believed that the presentation as nodal or extranodal involvement reflects the specific tissue "homing instincts" of the neoplastic cells.

Clinical features

There are three major clinical presentations:

1 *Extranodal.* These are tumors of adults and usually involve glandular tissues, most commonly the gastric mucosa where it has been associated with *Helicobacter pylori* gastritis. These latter cases are generally treated with antibiotics often leading to elimination of the organism and cure of the lymphoma. There is evidence that cases with the chromosal translocation t(11;18) will be resistant to antibiotic therapy. The pathologist may be able to predict these cases and those with a t(1;14)

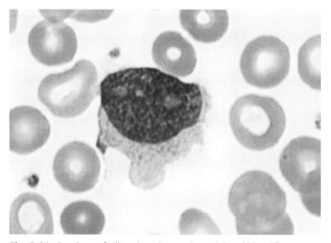

Fig. 8.61 Cytology of villous lymphocyte in peripheral blood from typical case of splenic lymphoma. Giemsa.

which also tend to be more aggressive by demonstrating abnormal bcl10 immunostaining in the nucleus of the lymphoma cells.[1,2] The disease is often localized with radiotherapy, often being highly successful in those cases refractory to antibiotic therapy. The clinical course is generally indolent and disseminated disease (e.g. to the bone marrow) is unusual at presentation and, as with other low-grade non-Hodgkin lymphomas (NHL), is not currently curable. Because the usual association is with glandular tissue, the majority of these extranodal marginal zone lymphomas are referred to as MALT lymphomas (or MALTomas).

2 *Splenic.* The exact relationship of splenic marginal zone lymphoma to the other marginal zone lymphomas remains unclear. It is now known to be sufficiently distinct to warrant a separate section in the WHO classification. This condition is probably what hematologists know as splenic lymphoma with circulating villous lymphocytes (Fig. 8.61).

3 *Nodal.* These cases represent primary nodal B cell neoplasms and there is no extranodal disease. Nodes involved by marginal zone lymphoma in patients with MALT lymphoma should be considered secondary to involvement rather than representing primary nodal disease. Occasionally, the disease is restricted to lymph nodes with or without bone marrow involvement.

Histopathology of the bone marrow

Marginal zone lymphomas: extranodal and nodal

Involvement of the bone marrow seems to be relatively uncommon (certainly less than 20% of cases) so that descriptions in the literature are of individual cases rather than series. The most common pattern is either the presence of central nodules or a patchy more diffuse infiltrate (Fig. 8.62).

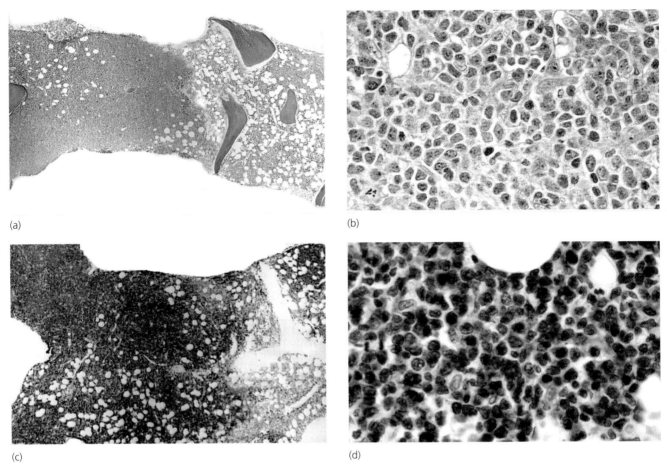

Fig. 8.62 MALT (mucosa-associated lymphoid tissue) lymphoma in the bone marrow. (a,b) Giemsa. (c,d) CD79 (B cell) immunostain.

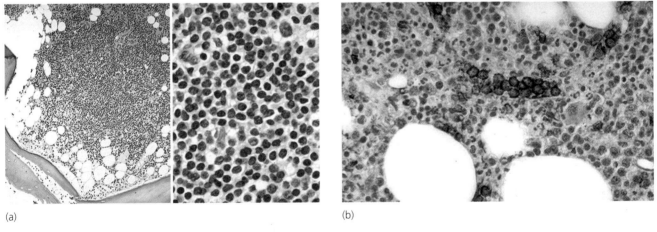

Fig. 8.63 Splenic lymphoma involving the bone marrow. (a) H&E. (b) CD20 (B cell immunostain).

Splenic marginal zone lymphoma

Most of these cases have involvement of the bone marrow. The most common pattern is similar to marginal zone lymphomas (i.e. with central nodules), although cases have been described that are entirely diffuse, some of which show plasmacytic differentiation with Dutcher bodies. Whether these latter cases have a relationship to lymphoplasmacytic lymphoma is unclear (Fig. 8.63) although a number of descriptions of typical Waldenström macroglobulinaemia in association with each of the three types of marginal zone lymphoma supports that relationship.[3]

Immunophenotype: IgM, IgD, CD19+, CD20+, CD22+, CD79+, CD43+/–, CD5–, CD10–, CD23–

Diagnostic problems

These are uncommon lesions with the bone marrow that are usually requested purely for staging purposes. The histology of the bone marrow alone is not diagnostic and by itself would probably be difficult to separate from some other similar B cell lymphomas such as lymphoplasmacytic lymphoma.

Key points

- Marginal zone lymphomas are mainly comprised of MALT lesions and their extensions into lymph nodes and other tissues.
- MALT lesions tend not to involve bone marrow (<20% of cases) unlike splenic marginal zone lymphomas where marrow infiltration is common.
- Splenic marginal zone lymphoma is distinct clinically from the other two types of marginal zone lymphoma.

References

1 Maes B, Demunter A, Peeters B, *et al.* bcl10 mutation does not represent an important pathogenic mechanism in gastric MALT-type lymphoma, and the presence of the API2-MLT fusion is associated with aberrant nuclear bcl10 expression. *Blood* 2002; **99**: 1398–404.

2 Ye H, Dogan A, Karran L, *et al.* bcl10 expression in normal and neoplastic lymphoid tissue. Nuclear localization in MALT lymphoma. *Am J Pathol* 2000; **157**: 1147–54.

3 Lin P, Hao S, Handy BC, *et al.* Lymphoid neoplasms associated with IgM paraprotein: a study of 382 patients. *Am J Clin Pathol* 2005; **123**: 200–5.

Chapter 8.8 Hairy cell leukemia

Hairy cell leukemia (HCL) was originally described as leukemic reticuloendotheliosis. Its current terminology is inspired by the hair-like processes of the leukemic cells seen with phase contrast or electron microscopy. HCL is a low-grade lymphoproliferative disorder of B lymphocytes which is now recognized as a distinct clinicopathologic entity.

Clinical features

The typical clinical picture is illustrated in Fig. 8.64.

Histopathology of the bone marrow

The cells are small (their nuclei being slightly larger than a resting lymphocyte) and lie spaced apart. The nuclei are oval or "bean" shaped, have one or two small inconspicuous nucleoli and are surrounded by a clear zone of cytoplasm (Fig. 8.65). The so-called hairs seen in smears and by electron microscopy are not apparent in conventional tissue sections (Fig. 8.66). Mitotic figures are rare.

A reticulin stain reveals fine fibrils distributed throughout the infiltrate, being present around almost every individual neoplastic cell. It is this extensive intercellular network of reticulin that is responsible for the "dry tap" during aspiration biopsy. There is no fibrosis (i.e. collagen production) (Fig. 8.67).

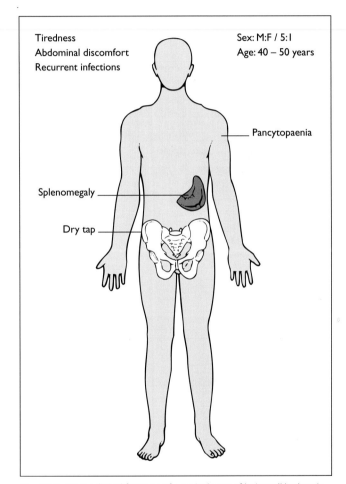

Tiredness
Abdominal discomfort
Recurrent infections

Sex: M:F / 5:1
Age: 40 – 50 years

Pancytopaenia

Splenomegaly

Dry tap

Fig. 8.64 Major clinical features of a typical case of hairy cell leukemia.

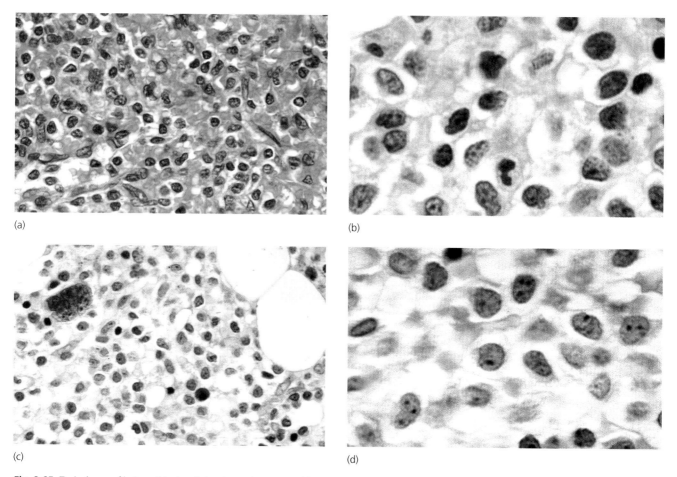

(a)

(b)

(c)

(d)

Fig. 8.65 Typical case of hairy cell leukemia in a bone marrow trephine. (a,b) H&E, medium and high power. (c,d) Giemsa, medium and high power.

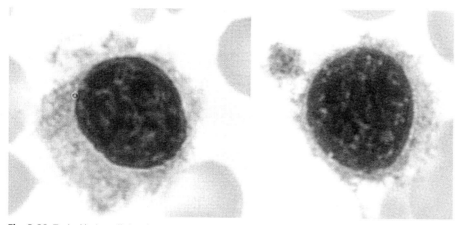

Fig. 8.66 Typical hairy cells in a bone marrow smear. Giemsa.

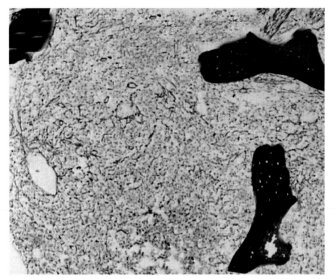

Fig. 8.67 Reticulin stain showing the fine fibrillar meshwork in a bone marrow infiltrated by hairy cell leukemia.

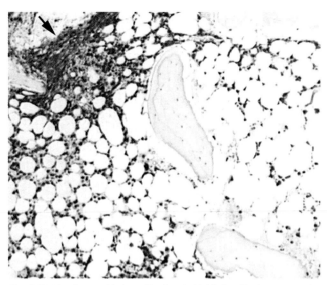

Fig. 8.68 Focal area of hairy cell leukemia highlighted by immunostaining for DBA.44 (arrow).

Patterns of involvement

The marrow is usually hypercellular. There are three main patterns of involvement by the neoplastic cells. All three patterns are often seen in the same specimen which is best appreciated by immunostaining.

1 *Focal involvement.* This is the most common pattern with the neoplastic cells forming ill-defined groups interspersed with normal hematopoietic tissue. This type of distribution means that a single trephine biopsy may sample an unaffected area, missing the main foci of disease. If the diagnosis is considered, hairy cells can be demonstrated by immunostaining in more than 95% of cases. Useful reagents are antibodies DBA.44 which probably belongs to CD75s (ex CDw76) (Fig. 8.68) and TRAP (tartrate-resistant acid phosphatase) which are reliable markers of hairy cells in fixed specimens.

2 *Diffuse involvement.* The hairy cells are dispersed throughout the marrow. This may range from a sparse infiltrate, easily overlooked, to virtual replacement of the marrow (Fig. 8.69).

3 *Interstitial involvement.* This is less common and refers to the presence of hairy cells lying amongst fat spaces in a hypoplastic marrow. In the absence of clinical suspicion they may be overlooked and a misdiagnosis of aplastic anemia made (Fig. 8.70).

A useful diagnostic feature is that low-power observation of the involved trephine biopsy will often show focal areas of hemorrhage within the marrow. These are equivalent to the "blood lakes" seen in sections of spleen involved by HCL (Fig. 8.71).

Hairy cells are unique B cells that coexpress many histiocytic antigens—a combination that is virtually diagnostic. For the fixed embedded trephine, positivity with the B cell antigens CD79a and CD20, combined with staining for CD68, TRAP and DBA.44, are a great assistance in establishing the diagnosis (Fig. 8.72).[1] One should also be aware that a certain proportion of cases are also positive for CD10 (apparently very common in Japan) and cyclin D1 (Fig. 8.73).[2-4] Most if not all cases are positive for CD25 although this is also expressed by many other lymphomas.

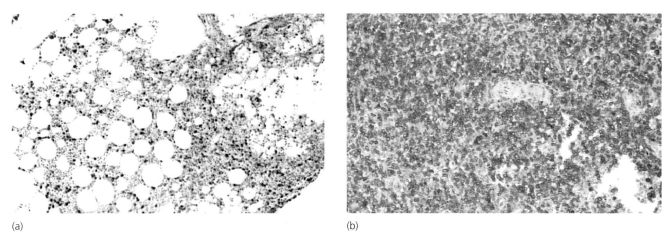

(a)

(b)

Fig. 8.69 Diffuse infiltration, both sparse (a) and heavy (b), of bone marrow by hairy cells highlighted by immunostaining for (a) DBA.44, (b) CD79a.

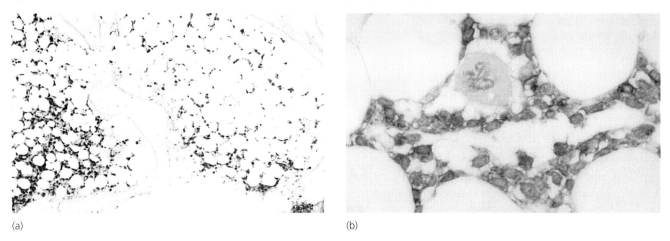

(a)

(b)

Fig. 8.70 Interstitial involvement of hypocellular bone marrow by hairy cells. (a,b) Low and high power immunostaining for DBA.44.

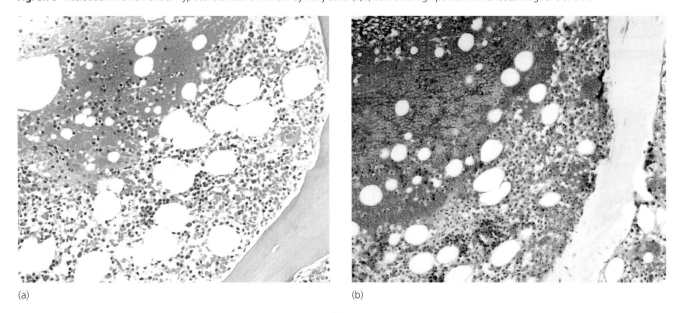

(a)

(b)

Fig. 8.71 "Blood lakes" in hairy cell leukemia. (a) H&E. (b) Immunostain for red cell glycophorin C.

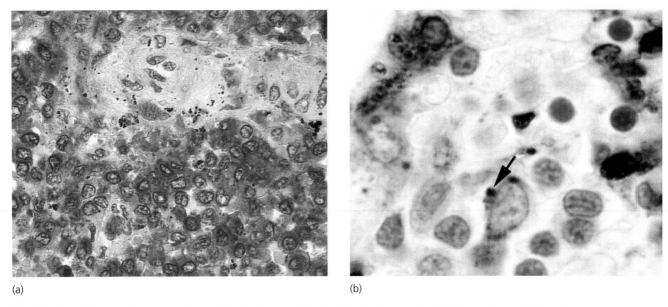

(a)   (b)

Fig. 8.72 Typical immunophenotype of hairy cell leukemia (a) positive for a B cell antigen such as CD79a combined with (b) cytoplasmic dot-positivity for CD68 (arrow). Positive staining for DBA.44 as illustrated earlier is also helpful.

CD10   cyclin D1

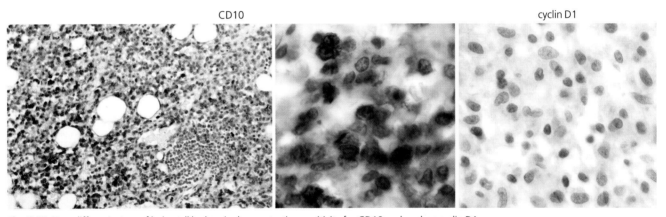

Fig. 8.73 Two different cases of hairy cell leukemia demonstrating positivity for CD10 and nuclear cyclin D1

Diagnostic problems

Differential diagnosis

In some cases of HCL the non-neoplastic marrow may show marked hyperplastic or even myelodysplastic features. If the hairy cell infiltrate is overlooked a misdiagnosis may be made (Fig. 8.74). Similarly, in hypocellular cases the sparse diffuse infiltrate is easily overlooked as consisting of erythroid precursors. It is easy to say the pathologist should have a high index of suspicion for all of these cases but we need some guidance clinically to do this. Conversely, if there is any clinical indication that HCL may be present only reject the diagnosis after exhausting all of the tests mentioned here (and even

then it might be wise to request another biopsy).

On occasion, other infiltrates may mimic HCL (e.g. mesenchymal chondroblastoma[5] and systemic mast cell disease[6]).

Assessing extent of marrow involvement

The extent of marrow involvement by hairy cells is often requested by clinicians as it allows an estimation to be made of the tumor load response to treatment. Complex semi-quantitative procedures have been described in the literature but have not been widely adopted by pathologists. At the present time a reasonable compromise would seem to be a low-power estimate of percentage marrow involved based on immunostaining for hairy cells.

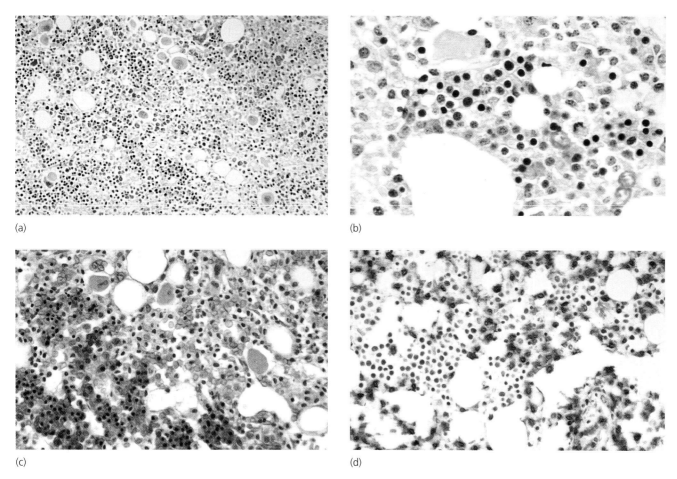

(a)

(b)

(c)

(d)

Fig. 8.74 Hypercellular bone marrow with marked erythroid hyperplasia. (a,b) Giemsa. (c) Immunostain for red cell glycophorin C, which is masking the underlying infiltrate of hairy cell leukemia. (d) Immunostain for B cell antigen, CD79a.

Assessing remission

Many patients with HCL in clinical remission show small numbers of hairy cells in their marrows, especially after immunocytochemical examination. The significance and clinical relevance of such residual disease remains unclear. This has led some authorities to allow the marrow to contain small numbers of hairy cells and still qualify as complete remission (Fig. 8.75).[7]

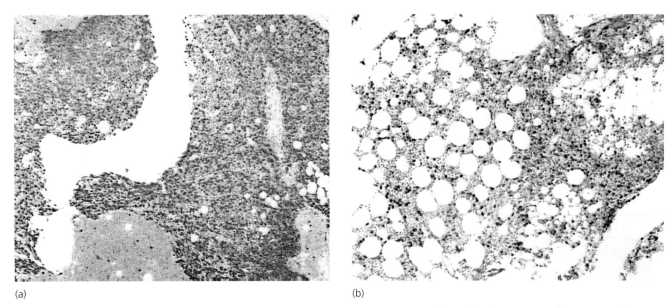

(a)   (b)

Fig. 8.75 Bone marrow in "remission" after treatment for hairy cell leukemia still contains an infiltrate when immunostained for DBA.44. (a) Pre-treatment. (b) Post-treatment.

Immunophenotype: CD20+, CD22+, CD79+, DBA.44+, TRAP+, CD68+, CD25+, CD10−/+, cyclin D1+/−, CD5−, CD23−

Key points

- Marrow involvement by hairy cells may be subtle.
- Characteristic histologic features include:
  bean-shaped nuclei
  spaced apart distribution
  delicate intercellular reticulin
  interstitial hemorrhage.
- Immunocytochemistry is of value, particularly in cases displaying subtle forms of marrow involvement.

References

1 Went PT, Zimpfer A, Pehrs AC, *et al.* High specificity of combined TRAP and DBA.44 expression for hairy cell leukemia. *Am J Surg Pathol* 2005; **29**: 474–8.

2 Dunphy CH, Oza YV, Skelly ME. An otherwise typical case of non-Japanese hairy cell leukemia with CD10 and CDw75 expression: response to cladaribine phosphate. *J Clin Lab Anal* 1999; **13**: 141–4.

3 Jasionowski TM, Hartung L, *et al.* Analysis of CD10+ hairy cell leukemia. *Am J Clin Pathol* 2003; **120**: 228–35.

4 Miranda RN, Briggs RC, Kinney MC, *et al.* Immunohistochemical detection of cyclin D1 using optimized conditions is highly specific for mantle cell lymphoma and hairy cell leukemia. *Mod Pathol* 2000; **13**: 1308–14.

5 Yam LT, Phyliky RL, Li C-Y. Benign and neoplastic disorders simulating hairy cell leukaemia. *Semin Oncol* 1984; **11**: 353–61.

6 Webb TA, Li C-Y, Yam LT. Systemic mast cell disease: a clinical and haematopathologic study of 26 cases. *Cancer* 1982; **49**: 927–38.

7 Naeim F, Jacobs AD. Bone marrow changes in patients with hairy cell leukaemia treated by recombinant alpha-interferon. *Hum Pathol* 1985; **16**: 1200–5.

Chapter 8.9 Multiple myeloma

Multiple myeloma is a clinical entity caused by a malignant monoclonal proliferation of plasma cells within the bone marrow. It is characterized by the following:

1 Increased numbers of clonal plasma cells within the bone marrow (>10% of the nucleated cell population).

2 Lytic bone lesions.

3 The presence of an M (or paraprotein) band identified electrophoretically in serum or urine.

At least two of these three components must be present before a diagnosis of myeloma can be made.

Clinical features

The most common clinical features associated with myeloma are illustrated in Fig. 8.76.

The clinical course is typically a cycle of remission following chemotherapy with eventual relapse into high-grade disease that is resistant to further chemotherapy. An indolent form, known as smoldering myeloma, has been described.[1]

Histopathology of the bone marrow

The marrow is typically hypercellular (Fig. 8.77). The normal hematopoietic elements still remain but are overrun by neoplastic plasma cells. These are usually distributed throughout the marrow space and tend to be organized in irregular clusters or in peri-vascular multilayers (Fig. 8.78).

Abnormal forms (bi- or multinucleate and blast cells) are typically present but the neoplastic cells may be so well-differentiated as to be indistinguishable from normal reactive plasma cells (Fig. 8.79). Patient survival can be related to the plasma cell morphology (Fig. 8.80).[2] The histologic features that may be used to distinguish reactive plasmacytosis from multiple myeloma are described in Table 8.5.

None of these criteria is absolute. Some conditions produce a marked plasmacytosis that is purely reactive in nature (e.g. HIV infection and hepatitis) (Fig. 8.81).

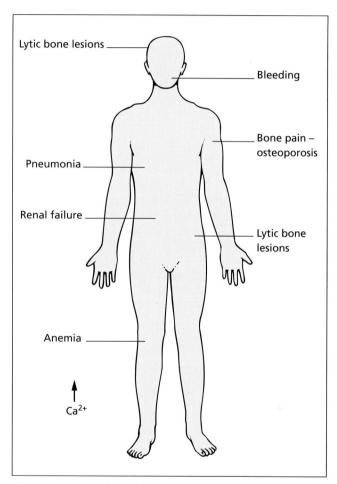

Fig. 8.76 Common clinical features in myeloma.

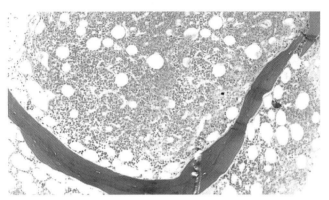

Fig. 8.77 Typical hypercellular bone marrow in myeloma. Giemsa.

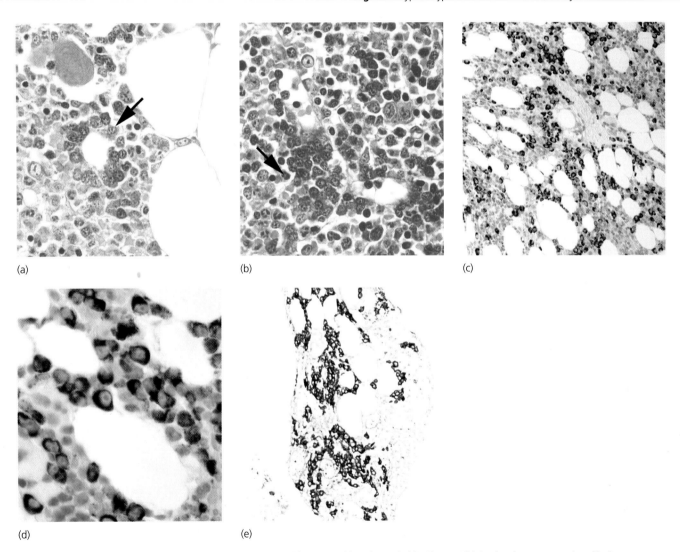

(a)

(b)

(c)

(d)

(e)

Fig. 8.78 Clustering of neoplastic plasma cells (arrows) around fat spaces (a) and vessels (b). Giemsa. This is often better appreciated by immunostaining with an antibody such as VS38 (p63) (c,d) or CD138 (e) which identify plasma cells.

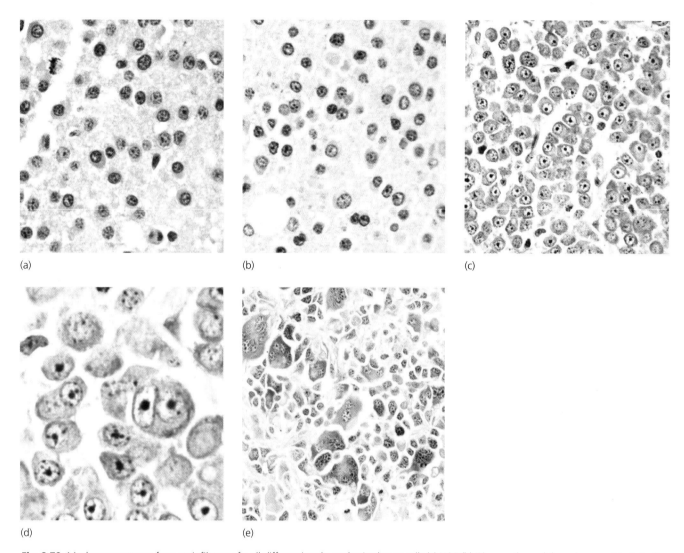

Fig. 8.79 Myeloma can range from an infiltrate of well-differentiated neoplastic plasma cells (a) H&E (b) Giemsa, through large immunoblasts (c,d) to frankly bizarre sarcoma-like blast cells (e) Giemsa.

Histologic groups	Main subtype	Survival (months)
Plasmacytic		
Marshalko		46
Small round		24
Small notched		19
Polymorphous		16
Plasmablastic		9

(a)

(b)

Fig. 8.80 (a) Range of differentiation of neoplastic plasma cells in myeloma and (b) their relationship to survival.

Table 8.5 A comparison of the histologic and immunophenotypic features of reactive plasmacytosis and multiple myeloma.

Reactive plasmacytosis	Multiple myeloma
Plasma cells usually constitute <25% of cells	Plasma cells usually constitute >25% of cells
Majority are mature plasma cells	Greater variation in size
Nucleoli only present in a few plasma cells	Nucleoli often present
Collections, i.e. nodules or sheets of plasma cells, never seen	Often present in large homogeneous groups
Occasional binucleated forms and less mature forms	Plasmablast forms (prominent central nucleoli)
Single layer around capillaries	Several cells deep around capillaries, diffusely distributed amongst fat cells, groups or sheets of plasma cells
Polyclonal light chains	Monoclonal light chains
CD56 negative	CD56 positive

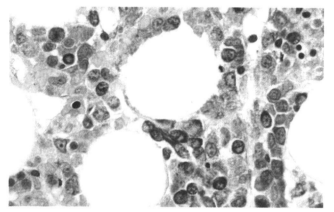

Fig. 8.81 Reactive plasmacytosis in HIV infection.

Immunophenotype

Although most plasma cells lack CD20 approximately one-third of myeloma cases express this antigen (Fig. 8.82) along with CD79a, CD38, VS38 (p63) and CD138 (syndecan). Neoplastic plasma cells often express CD56 (Fig. 8.83)[3] whereas reactive ones do not. However, the only certain means of separating the two conditions is by demonstrating monoclonality. This is most easily carried out immunohisto-chemically by showing the presence of light chain restriction.

Reactive plasma cells will have a ratio of about two λ positive cells to every κ positive cell. In contrast, myeloma cells will all belong to the same clone and secrete only one type of light chain. There are always some reactive plasma cells mixed in with the myeloma cells so in practice monoclonality is identified by a ratio outside the normal 2 : 1. Typically, a ratio of 10 : 1 of κ to λ or 5 : 1 if λ is the dominant type provides evidence for the neoplastic nature of the plasma cells (Fig. 8.84).

On a practical note, one should be reluctant to accept immunostaining as reliable if all the plasma cells are negative for one of the light chains (there should be a few positive reactive plasma cells), because this is more likely to indicate technical failure rather than an exclusive type of light chain production. This is especially important if not all of the plasma cells are positive for the other chain. Occasionally for technical reasons it is not possible to achieve good light chain immunostaining. In these cases *in situ* hybridization for light chain RNA can be diagnostic.

Myeloma cells are another example of hematopoietic tumors expressing cyclin D1 (Fig. 8.85) and indeed there is evidence that positive cases have a worse prognosis.[4] It is believed that myelomas with a higher proliferation rate (assessed by antibodies such as Ki67) also do worse.[5,6]

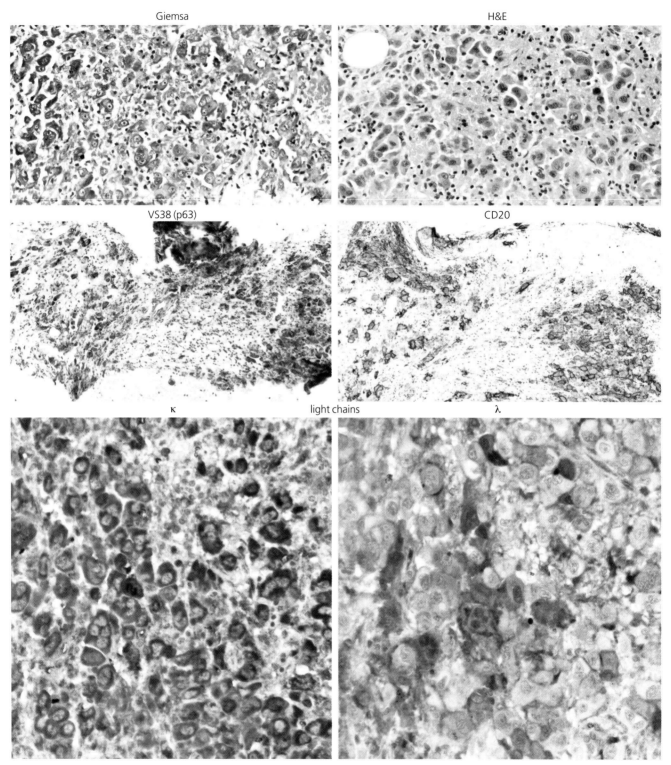

Fig. 8.82 CD20 positive case of myeloma with otherwise typical histology and immunophenotype.

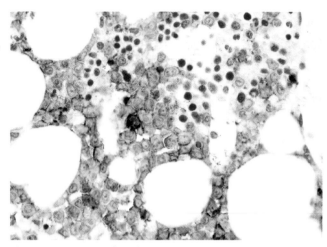

Fig. 8.83 Most cases of myeloma express CD56 at least partially.

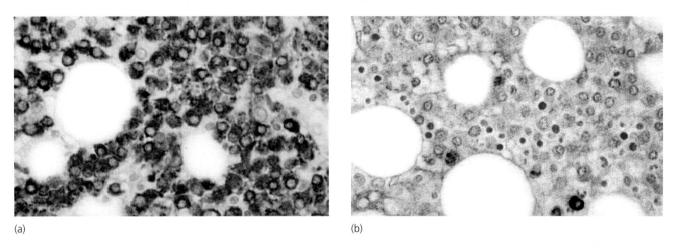

(a)

(b)

Fig. 8.84 Light chain restriction in myeloma. λ Positive myeloma cells (a) greatly outnumber a few remaining benign κ positive cells (b).

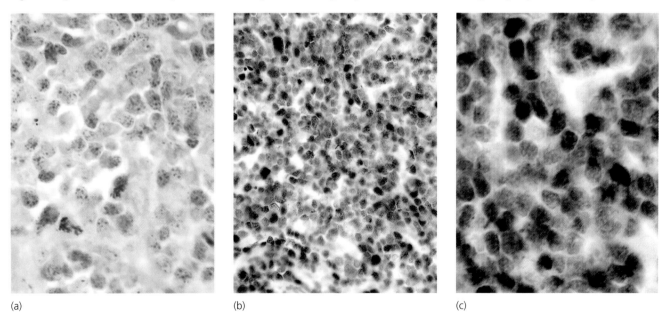

(a)

(b)

(c)

Fig. 8.85 Many cases of myeloma express nuclear cyclin D1. (a) Giemsa, (b) and (c) cyclin D1.

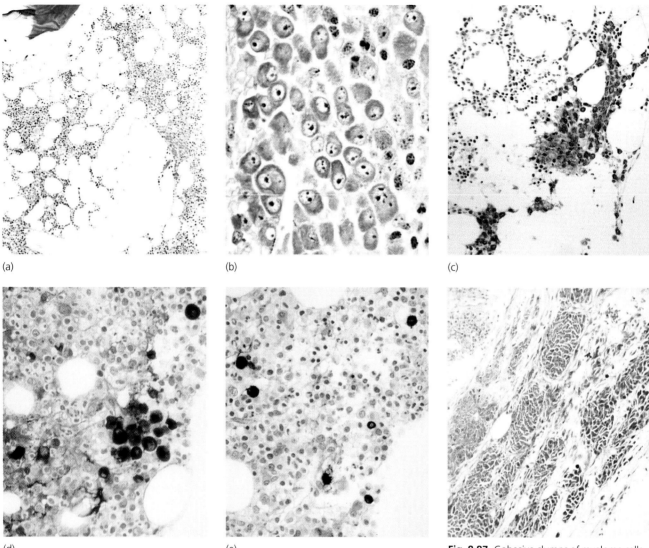

(a)

(b)

(c)

(d)

(e)

Fig. 8.87 Cohesive clumps of myeloma cells mimicking metastatic carcinoma.

Fig. 8.86 Focal infiltration of myeloma. (a,b) Giemsa. (c) VS38 immunostain for plasma cells. (d) λ and (e) κ light chain immunostains.

Immunophenotype: CD20–/+, CD79+, CD38+, CD56+, CD138+, VS38+, cyclin D1–/+, monoclonal light chains

Less common appearances

1 Myeloma cells can be inconspicuous when they are present in small numbers and infiltrate the marrow diffusely without any clustering.
2 The infiltration may be focal and not aspirated (Fig. 8.86).
3 Myeloma cells may form cohesive groups which can be mistaken for metastatic disease such as breast cancer (Fig. 8.87).

4 The myeloma cells may have a vacuolated cytoplasm (Mott cells) which can be misidentified as histiocytes or mucus-producing cells (Fig. 8.88).
5 The myeloma cells may have cleaved or multilobated nuclei which may resemble other lymphomas and leukemias or even some non-hematopoietic tumors.

In all of these situations the most valuable diagnostic aid is light chain immunostaining.

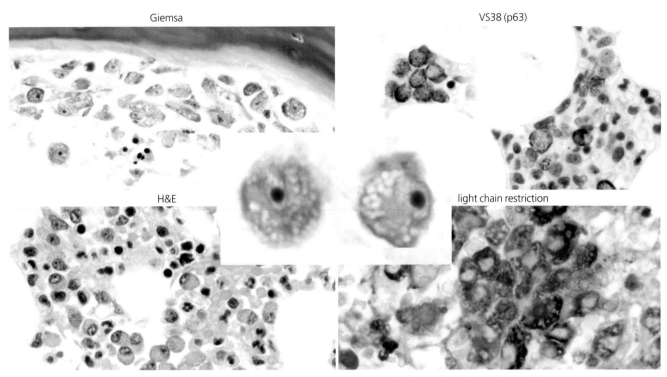

Fig. 8.88 Mott cell myeloma demonstrating typical appearances with Giemsa (low and high power) and H&E. These cells have a typical immunophenotype illustrated here by VS38 and light chain restriction.

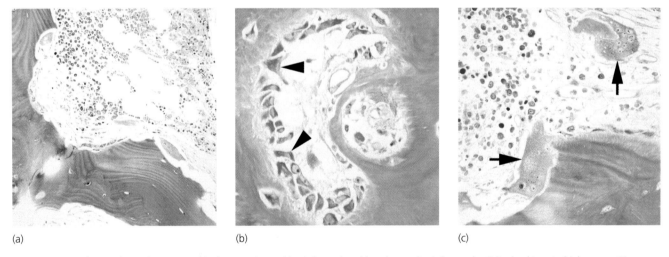

(a)   (b)   (c)

Fig. 8.89 Bone changes in myeloma caused by increased osteoblastic (arrowheads) and osteoclastic (arrows) activity. (a–c) Low to high power. Giemsa.

Other features occasionally seen in association with myeloma

1 Destruction of the bone by osteoclasts causing the characteristic lytic lesions in myeloma. The neoplastic plasma cells themselves do not resorb bone (Fig. 8.89).

2 The secretion of light chains by the myeloma cells can lead to the deposition of amyloid within the marrow (Fig. 8.90).

3 About 10% of myeloma cases will have increased reticulin staining and hence a trephine biopsy is more likely to be diagnostic than an aspirate (Fig. 8.91).

4 The presence of sarcoid-like granulomas occurs occasionally in myeloma. Its significance is unclear (Fig. 8.92).[7]

5 Multiple reactive lymphoid aggregates (less than three per low-power field) may be found in a minority of cases and are said to be associated with fewer lytic bone lesions.[8]

6 Other malignancies such as chronic myeloproliferative disorders and acute leukemias may be found coexisting with myeloma in the marrow.

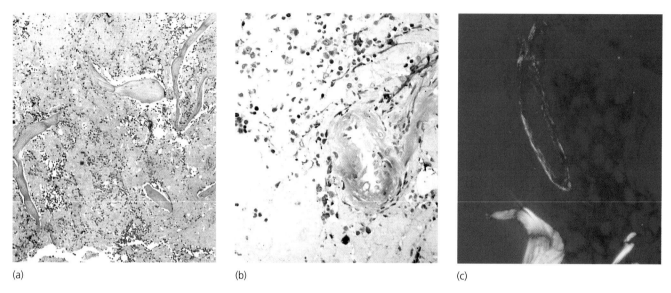

Fig. 8.90 Amyloid deposition in myeloma. (a) H&E. (b) Giemsa. (c) Congo red.

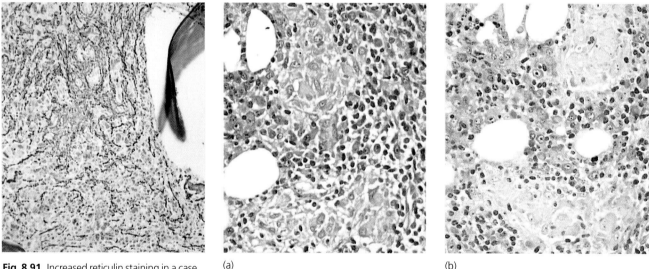

Fig. 8.91 Increased reticulin staining in a case of myeloma.

Fig. 8.92 Granuloma formation associated with myeloma. (a) H&E. (b) Giemsa.

Diagnostic problems

What is the significance of a low number of monoclonal plasma cells in a marrow?

The detection of a neoplastic population of plasma cells in a marrow, where the full criteria for multiple myeloma are not met, probably reflects our ability to detect the disease at an earlier stage in its development than had been possible before the introduction of immunohistochemical techniques. A small number of asymptomatic individuals (usually elderly) in the population have a monoclonal band in their serum. This is not of light chain type, as is usually the case in myeloma, but is immunoglobulin G (IgG) or IgM. The neoplastic clone secreting this paraprotein is usually too small to detect in bone marrow biopsies. These cases have been called monoclonal gammopathy of uncertain significance (MGUS) or benign paraproteinemia. While some cases (about 30% over a 10-year period) progress to myelomatosis the majority appear to remain healthy. Thus, detection of a plasma cell monoclone in the marrow is not *per se* definite evidence of incipient myeloma. Obviously, such individuals will require careful monitoring.

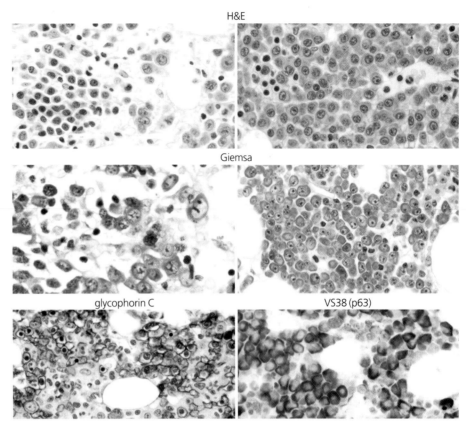

Fig. 8.93 Erythroblasts (left column) resemble plasmablasts (right column) by H&E staining but are more easily identified by Giemsa or immunostaining for red cell antigens such as glycophorin C (compared with plasma cell antigens such as VS38).

What other cells resemble plasma cells?

Erythroblasts

Plasmablasts may resemble erythroblasts, because both cell types possess a paranuclear hof. This is especially apparent in H&E-stained sections, whereas Giemsa staining reveals a delicate blue in erythroid cytoplasm contrasting with the lilac hue of the plasmablast (Fig. 8.93).

In addition, the plasmablast has a single nucleolus while the erythroblast usually has more than one. Groups of erythroblasts are often found in association with more mature, and therefore more readily identified, elements such as normoblasts. Unequivocal evidence of a cell's nature is provided by immunohistochemistry for erythroid and lymphoid markers.

Promyelocytes

The promyelocytes of acute promyelocytic leukemia may resemble plasma cells as their nucleus is eccentrically placed and their cytoplasm plentiful. The chromatin pattern is quite different because the promyelocyte's nucleus is densely staining and lacks the plasma cell's "clock face" nucleus or the plasmablast's prominent solitary nucleolus. Immunohistochemistry will easily resolve those cases where doubt remains (Fig. 8.94).

Osteoblasts

Although it is unlikely to be a source of diagnostic difficulty, it should be remembered that osteoblasts morphologically resemble plasma cells. Their distinctive paratrabecular distribution readily identifies their true nature (Fig. 8.95).

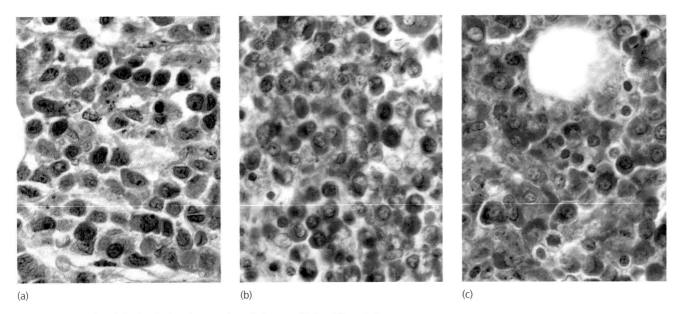

(a) (b) (c)

Fig. 8.94 Promyelocytic leukemia showing prominent "plasma cell"-like differentiation.

Key points

- Immunohistochemistry is invaluable in separating reactive plasmacytosis from multiple myeloma and in identifying cases of "early" myeloma where the number of plasma cells is low.
- The degree of plasma cell differentiation and pattern of marrow involvement may relate to prognosis.
- While most cases of myeloma are diagnostically straightforward, a few cases will involve the marrow more subtly. Careful inspection of the marrow section and the use of immunocytochemistry will reveal them.

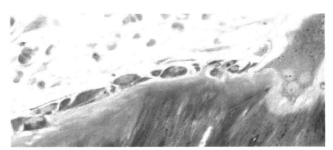

Fig. 8.95 Osteoblasts may look remarkably like plasma cells but are readily identified by their paratrabecular location.

References

1 Kyle RA, Greipp PR. Smoldering multiple myeloma. *N Engl J Med* 1980; **302**: 1347–9.

2 Bartl R, Frisch B. Bone marrow histology in multiple myeloma: prognostic relevance of histologic characteristics. *Haematol Rev* 1989; **3**: 87–108.

3 Van Camp B, Durie B, Spier C, *et al.* Plasma cells in multiple myeloma express a natural killer cell-associated antigen: CD56 (NHK-1; Leu-19). *Blood* 1990; **76**: 377–82.

4 Hoechtlen-Vollmar W, Menzel G, Bartl R, *et al.* Amplification of cyclin D1 gene in multiple myeloma: clinical and prognostic relevance. *Br J Haematol* 2000; **109**: 30.

5 Barlogie B, Epstein J, Selvanayagam P, *et al.* Plasma cell myeloma: new biological insights and advances in therapy. *Blood* 1989; **73**: 865–79.

6 Kanavaros P, Stefanaki K, Vlachonikolis J, *et al.* Immunohistochemical expression of the p53, p21/Waf-1, Rb, p16 and Ki67 proteins in multiple myeloma. *Anticancer Res* 2000; **20(6B)**: 4619–25.

7 Falini B, Tabilio A, Veelardi A, *et al.* Multiple myeloma with a sarcoidosis-like reaction. *Scand J Haematol* 1982; **29**: 211–6.

8 Aghai E, Avni G, Lurie M, *et al.* Bone marrow biopsy in multiple myeloma: a clinical pathological study. *Isr J Med Sci* 1988; **24**: 298–301.

Chapter 8.10 Diffuse large B cell lymphoma

Within the WHO classification, this entity encompasses a number of conditions described by Kiel and other groups. These include centroblastic, immunoblastic and T-cell-rich B cell lymphoma. This is because even experienced pathologists have great difficulty in recognizing those subdivisions described to date (Fig. 8.96).

Large cell lymphomas with an anaplastic morphology are also currently included in this category and not as anaplastic large cell lymphomas. A further justification for a single grouping is that at present there is no firm evidence to suggest that the treatment or prognosis of any of these conditions differs (Fig. 8.97). Recent genetic studies of diffuse large B cell lymphomas using DNA microarray technology have suggested that a division into those tumors arising from germinal center B cells and those from post germinal center or activated B cells is clinically significant with the former having a better overall survival. It may be possible to make this distinction immunocytochemically (see below) so the results of follow-up studies on these findings are eagerly awaited.[1-3]

Diffuse large B cell lymphomas constitute about 40% of adult NHL. Most patients are over 40 years old and present with rapidly enlarging lymph nodes although a substantial minority of cases will be extranodal. It is an aggressive but potentially curable condition.

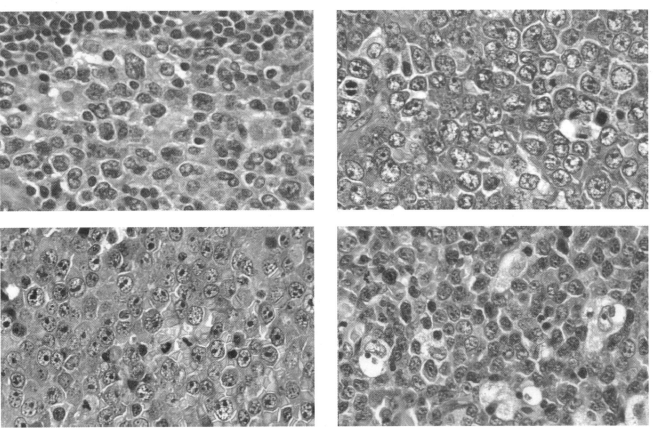

Fig. 8.96 Four different large B cell lymphomas illustrating the cellular heterogeneity of this category.

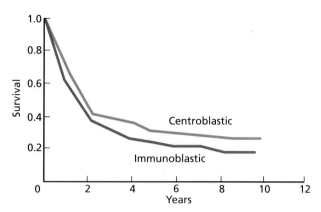

Fig. 8.97 Survival curve of centroblastic and immunoblastic lymphomas diagnosed by Kiel criteria.

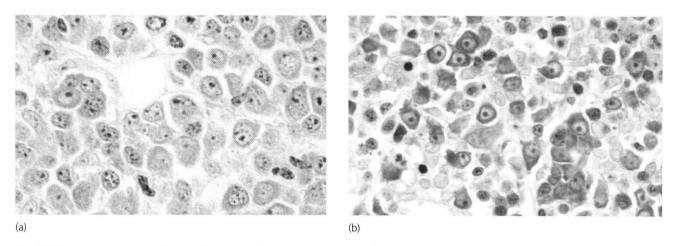

(a)   (b)

Fig. 8.98 Two typical examples of large cell lymphoma in the bone marrow. Note the high degree of cellular heterogeneity. Giemsa.

> *Immunophenotype germinal center type:* surface Ig+/–, CD19+, CD20+, CD22+, CD79a+, bcl6+, CD10+, CD5–/+, CD45+/–, bcl2–
> *Immunophenotype activated B cell-like type:* surface Ig+/–, CD19+, CD20+, CD22+, CD79a+, bcl6–, CD10–, CD5+/–, CD45+/–, bcl2+

Histopathology of the bone marrow

The neoplastic cells have large vesicular nuclei, prominent nucleoli, basophilic cytoplasm and easily found mitotic figures. There is variability in the morphology of these large cells which gave rise to their description as separate categories in other classifications. In practice these lymphomas usually have a heterogeneous cell population which has made for high intra- and interobserver error in classification (Fig. 8.98).

Immunophenotypically they are virtually all CD20 positive (hence the value of rituximab in therapy) (Fig. 8.99) and for other pan-B cell markers such as CD79a and PAX5. As mentioned above, there is a growing consensus that a division into germinal center B (GCB) and activated B-cell-like (ABC) diffuse large B cell lymphomas will prove useful. It has been suggested that this distinction can be made immunocytochemically with GCB being CD10+ bcl6+ and bcl2–, whereas ABC are CD10–, bcl6– and bcl2+. Other markers when expressed that have been linked with a poorer prognosis are CD5, p53, Ki67 and CD44.[3] None of these produce clearly defined groups and all have a high degree of overlap so there is as yet no conclusive evidence for their implementation in diagnostic practice.

Table 8.6 Differential diagnosis of anaplastic lymphomas.

Antibody	Large cell anaplastic morphology*	Other large cell	Carcinoma
CD45	–/+	+	–
CD30	+/–	–/+	–
CD20/PAX5	+	+	–
CD3	–	–	–
Anti-cytokeratins	–	–	+
EMA	–/+	–	+/–

*These B cell cases are classified as large cell lymphomas not anaplastic lymphomas in the WHO scheme.

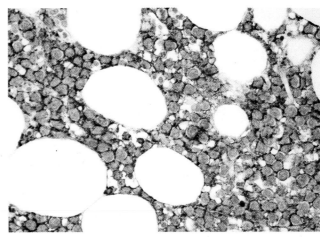

Fig. 8.99 Diffuse large B cell lymphomas are virtually all strongly CD20 positive.

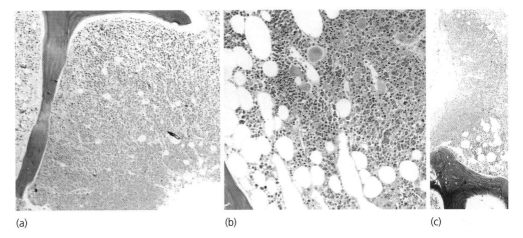

(a) (b) (c)

Fig. 8.100 Different patterns of involvement of the bone marrow by large cell lymphoma. Giemsa.

When present, involvement of bone marrow is usually obvious but without any particular histologic pattern (Fig. 8.100). Occasionally, large B cell lymphomas consist only of scattered malignant cells with a florid T cell reaction known as T-cell-rich B cell lymphomas (Fig. 8.101). A rare variant easily missed on morphology alone is the intravascular large cell lymphoma previously known as "malignant angioendotheliosis" (Fig. 8.102).

Diagnostic problems

Diffuse large B cell lymphoma vs. anaplastic carcinoma

It is important to make the distinction between these two groups because the treatment regimens differ and a cure is more likely in the lymphoma group if appropriate treatment is given. Distinction is possible immunohistochemically (Fig. 8.103).

In those cases with an anaplastic large cell morphology, the resemblance to metastatic carcinoma can be strong. The antibodies shown in Table 8.6 will help in distinguishing between these groups.

Diffuse large B cell lymphoma vs. lymphoblastic lymphoma

Although this is usually straightforward based on cytology and positivity of lymphoblastic lymphoma for terminal deoxynucleotidyl transferase (TdT), rare cases of large B cell lymphoma, which otherwise do not look lymphoblastic, may express TdT (Fig. 8.104). At present in such a case the best one can do is reach a consensus diagnosis with the clinicians.

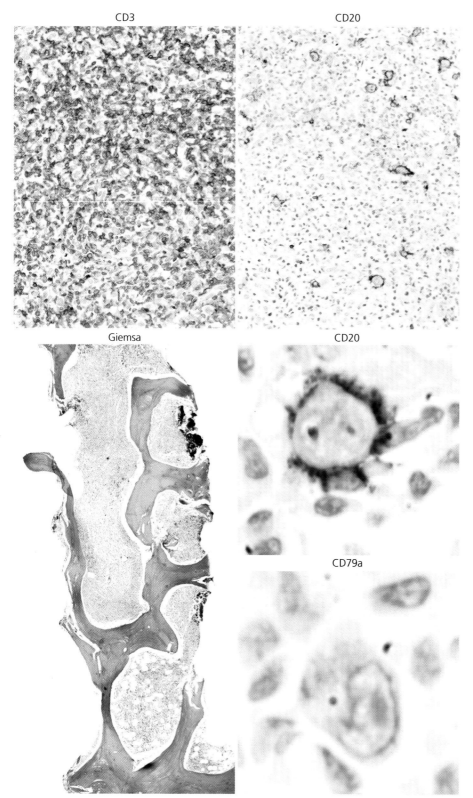

Fig. 8.101 T-cell-rich large B cell lymphoma in the bone marrow immunostained for CD3, CD20 and CD79a.

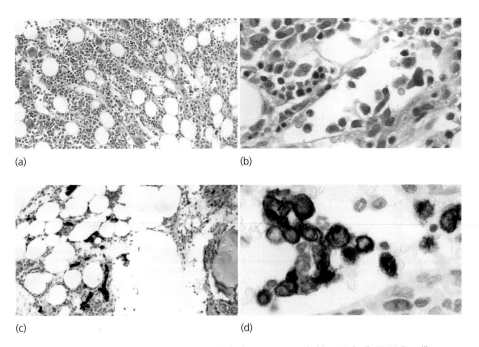

(a)

(b)

(c)

(d)

Fig. 8.102 Intravascular large cell lymphoma in the bone marrow. (a,b) H&E. (c,d) CD79 (B cell).

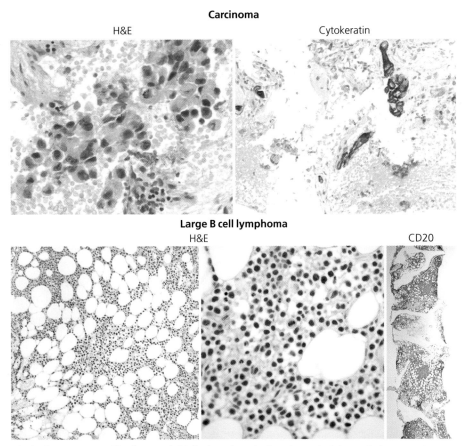

Carcinoma

H&E   Cytokeratin

Large B cell lymphoma

H&E   CD20

Fig. 8.103 Two cases with large cell infiltrates in the bone marrow. The first was initially thought to be lymphoma but shown to be secondary carcinoma by immunostaining for cytokeratins whereas the second was poorly fixed and mistaken for carcinoma but was actually a diffuse large B cell lymphoma on immunostaining.

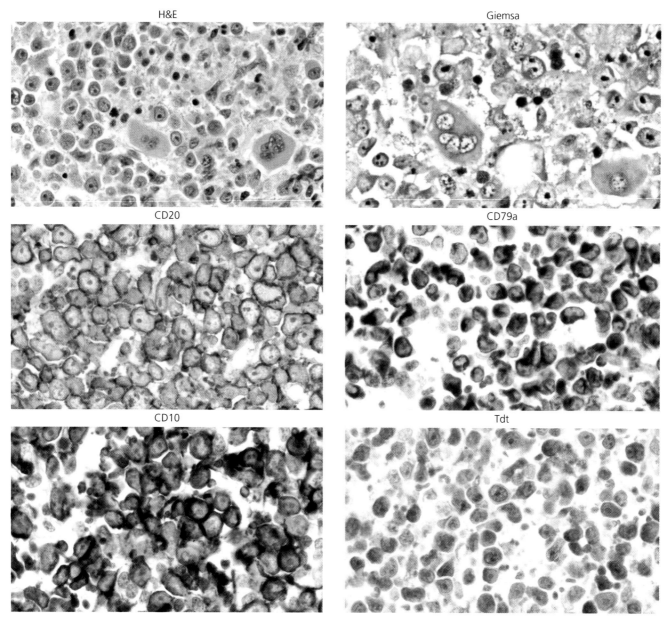

H&E

Giemsa

CD20

CD79a

CD10

Tdt

Fig. 8.104 Example of a diffuse large B cell lymphoma in bone marrow expressing terminal deoxynucleotidyl transferase (TdT). At least it looks like that and clinically the age and other features were against a lymphoblastic diagnosis.

Key points

- Diffuse large B cell lymphomas consist of several morphologic types.
- They are clinically aggressive but potentially curable.
- Distinction must be made from anaplastic carcinoma.

References

1 Alizadeh AA, Eisen MB, Davis RE, *et al*. Distinct types of diffuse large B-cell lymphoma identified by gene expression profiling. *Nature* 2000; **403**: 503–11.

2 Lossos IS, Czerwinski DK, Alizadeh AA, *et al*. Prediction of survival in diffuse large B-cell lymphoma based on the expression of six genes. *N Engl J Med* 2004; **350**: 1828–37.

3 Tzankov A, Pehrs AC, Zimpfer A, *et al*. Prognostic significance of CD44 expression in diffuse large B cell lymphoma of activated and germinal centre B cell-like types: a tissue microarray analysis of 90 cases. *J Clin Pathol* 2003; **56**: 747–52.

Chapter 8.11 Burkitt lymphoma

This lymphoma occurs in two different settings although the histologic appearances are identical. The African (endemic) form is the most common childhood (4–7 years) malignancy in parts of equatorial Africa and in New Guinea. The lymphoma tends to involve the jaw, either mandible or maxilla, and may extend up into the orbit. Other organs are commonly involved (e.g. ovary, testes, liver, retroperitoneum, breast and gastrointestinal tract). It is associated with Epstein–Barr virus (EBV) and involves a chromosomal translocation, commonly t(8;14).

The non-African (non-endemic) form is a rare lymphoma and occurs over a wider age range with many adult cases, often those with an immunodeficiency, and involves the gastrointestinal tract (particularly the terminal ileum),

ovaries and kidneys. Lymph node involvement is less frequently seen than in most other lymphomas. EBV is associated with a minority of these cases, usually those with immunodeficiency.

The genetic features suggest that the endemic form is a neoplasm involving an early B cell while the non-endemic form arises from a B cell at a later stage of development.

The lymphoma is highly aggressive, having the fastest doubling time of any known human neoplasm, although it is potentially curable.

The WHO classification has quietly dropped the apostrophe from the end of the name of this tumor which seems a relatively unimportant change. This text uses this new term but we would leave it to others to use whichever term they prefer.

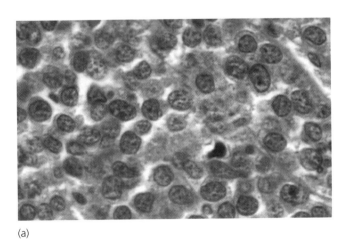

(a)

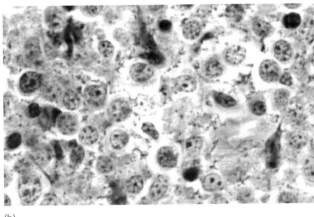

(b)

Fig. 8.105 Burkitt lymphoma cells in a bone marrow trephine. (a) H&E. (b) Giemsa.

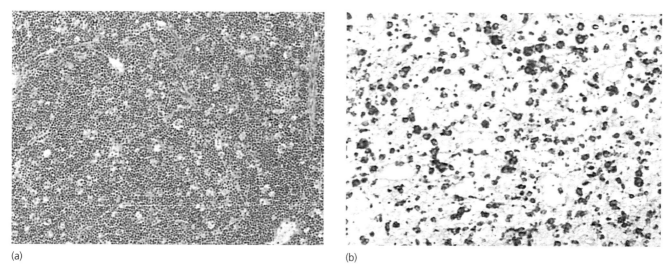

(a)

(b)

Fig. 8.106 Starry sky appearance of Burkitt lymphoma as seen in lymph nodes is uncommon in bone marrow sections. (a) H&E (ovary). (b) CD68 immunostain for macrophages.

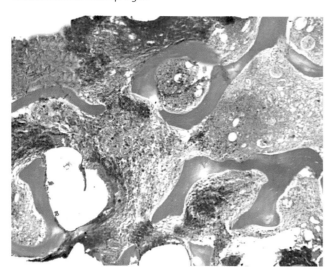

Fig. 8.107 Typical low power picture of Burkitt lymphoma in a bone marrow trephine.

Immunophenotype: SIgM+, CD19+, CD20+, CD22+, CD79a+, CD10+, bcl6+, CD5−, CD23−, TdT−, bcl2−, >95% proliferation fraction (Ki67)

Histopathology of the bone marrow

The marrow is involved in about 20% of non-endemic cases.

The neoplastic cell has the same appearance in both forms of the disease. It is a monomorphic medium-sized cell with a moderate amount of basophilic cytoplasm and a regular oval or round nucleus containing 2–5 small nucleoli (Fig. 8.105). Mitotic figures are numerous, although the "starry sky" appearance seen in other organs is not a feature (Fig. 8.106). Frank necrosis may be seen, particularly following chemotherapy. The marrow is usually hypercellular although interstitial, nodular and diffuse patterns of infiltration may occur (Fig. 8.107). The immunophenotype is very characteristic and usually assists in making a secure diagnosis (Fig. 8.108).

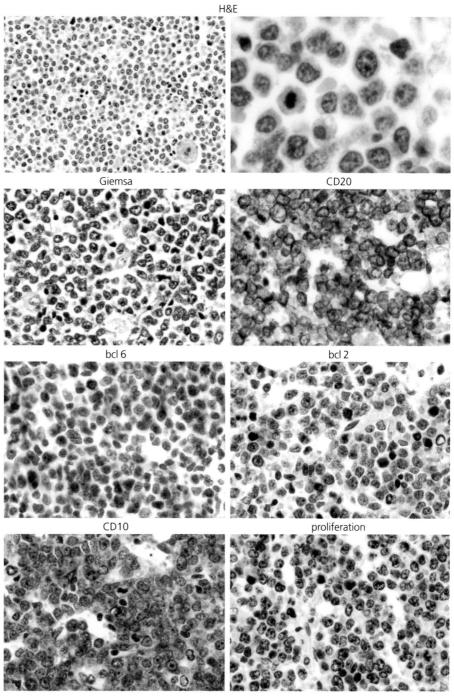

Fig. 8.108 Characteristic histology and immunostaining pattern of Burkitt lymphoma. Note that the bcl2 staining is negative although there are a few T cells around as an internal control and that the proliferation is close to 100% (Ki67).

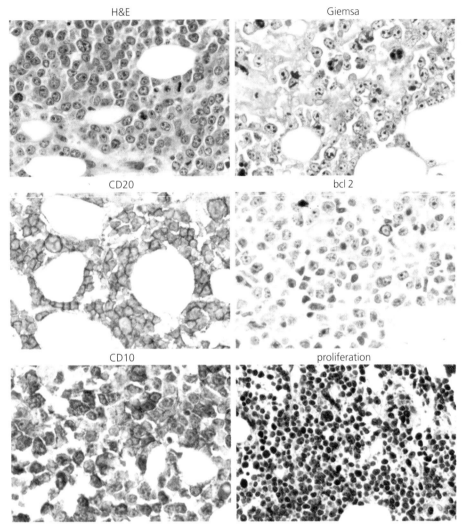

Fig. 8.109 A case of atypical Burkitt/Burkitt-like lymphoma where the morphology is suggestive of a large B cell lymphoma but the immunophenotype is characteristic of Burkitt lymphoma.

Diagnostic problems

Burkitt lymphoma vs. lymphoblastic lymphoma

Similarities exist between these two high-grade lymphomas; indeed, for some time the Kiel classification treated Burkitt lymphoma as a subtype of lymphoblastic lymphoma. Careful evaluation of the nuclear morphology, in particular the multiple nucleoli seen in Burkitt lymphoma, is useful in separating the two entities. This is not always as easy as some texts make out. It is often worth examining the figures in such texts and on putting one's thumb over the starry sky macrophage seeing if a difference can be perceived. Assessment of proliferation with antibodies such as Ki67 may be helpful because in Burkitt lymphoma all (or nearly all!) of the viable tumor cells will be positive (Fig. 8.108). In addition, Burkitt lymphoma cells do not express terminal deoxynucleotidyl transferase (TdT) or bcl2.

Burkitt lymphoma vs. anaplastic carcinoma

The relatively abundant cytoplasm of the lymphoma cells and their tendency to form "cohesive" clumps may impart an impression of carcinoma. Immunohistochemistry for lymphoid and epithelial markers will easily distinguish between the two diseases.

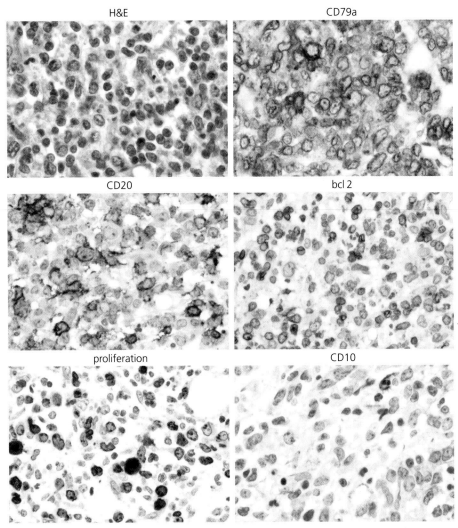

Fig. 8.110 In this case the morphology pointed towards Burkitt lymphoma but the immunophenotype favors a large B cell lymphoma with a moderate growth rate, positive bcl2 and negative CD10.

Burkitt lymphoma vs. large cell lymphoma

Occasional cases arise where it is difficult to distinguish between these two conditions. In these cases the neoplastic cells are more pleomorphic and larger than typical Burkitt lymphoma cells, with larger numbers of nucleoli. These cases have been categorized in the WHO classification as Burkitt lymphoma variant: atypical Burkitt/Burkitt-like (Fig 8.109). The immunophenotype remains that of typical Burkitt lymphoma so that if there are any deviations (e.g. less than 95% proliferation or bcl2 positivity) most experts would suggest a diagnosis of diffuse large B cell lymphoma (Fig. 8.110).

Necrotic tumors

Because of the phenomenal growth rate, Burkitt lymphomas are frequently necrotic. This causes severe problems with interpreting the histology but careful immunostaining will usually identify areas that are sufficiently preserved to enable the immunophenotype to be identified (Fig. 8.111).

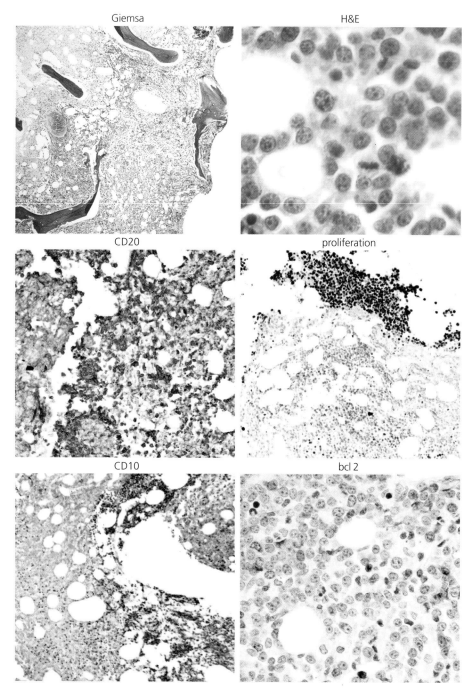

Giemsa

H&E

CD20

proliferation

CD10

bcl 2

Fig. 8.111 This is an example of Burkitt lymphoma in which most of the tumor is necrotic. However, there is, as illustrated, a small area of reasonably preserved histology which immunophenotypes characteristically. Note in particular that CD10 and CD20 are quite robust in staining even the most necrotic area whereas the proliferation marker Ki67 is restricted to the better preserved areas.

Key points

- Two forms exist: an endemic and a non-endemic. Although histologically identical, they have different clinical presentations.
- Very high proliferation rate as demonstrated by antibodies (e.g. Ki67 or mib-1).
- Immunohistochemistry will distinguish between anaplastic carcinoma and lymphoblastic lymphoma.

Chapter 8.12 Large granular lymphocyte leukemia

This is an uncommon condition also described as CD8 lymphocytosis with neutropenia or Tγ lymphoproliferative disease. The peripheral blood lymphocytosis is composed of cells with round or oval nuclei with moderately condensed chromatin and rare nucleoli, eccentrically placed in abundant pale blue cytoplasm with azurophilic granules (Fig. 8.112).

There are two major lineages: one being T cell and the other having a natural killer (NK) cell phenotype. Patients with the T cell phenotype show clonal rearrangement of the T cell receptor genes whereas these genes show germline configuration in the NK cell cases. T cell cases are predominantly a disease of late middle age and are associated with recurrent bacterial infections (a consequence of the invariable neutropenia). About 30% of patients have rheumatoid arthritis and Felty or a Felty-like syndrome. The clinical course is usually indolent.

NK cell cases are usually younger with more severe clinical symptoms of anemia and thrombocytopenia and more widespread tissue infiltration. Clonal cytogenetic abnormalities associated with Epstein–Barr virus infection have been reported in a number of clinically aggressive cases from Japan, East Asia and Central and South America.

Although debate continues whether large granular lymphocyte (LGL) proliferations are reactive or neoplastic, it is being progressively accepted as a leukemia based on the observations of clonality and tissue invasion by LGLs of marrow, spleen and liver.

Histopathology of the bone marrow

Bone marrow infiltration is usually sparse, with mild to moderate lymphocytosis as well as focal nodules composed of both B and T cells. A diagnosis is unlikely on the trephine alone, which can be easily misinterpreted as a B cell lymphoma (Fig. 8.113).

The key to the diagnosis is the peripheral blood smear which can be confirmed by flow cytometry or splenic histology if the spleen is removed (Fig. 8.114). There may be a myeloid maturation arrest or erythroid hypoplasia.

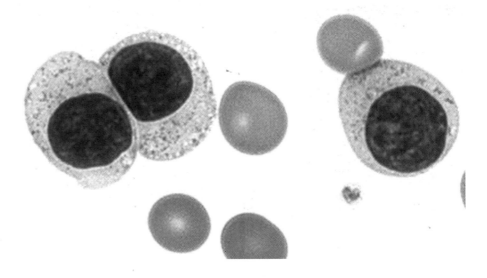

Fig. 8.112 The cytology of large granular lymphocytes (LGL) in peripheral blood.

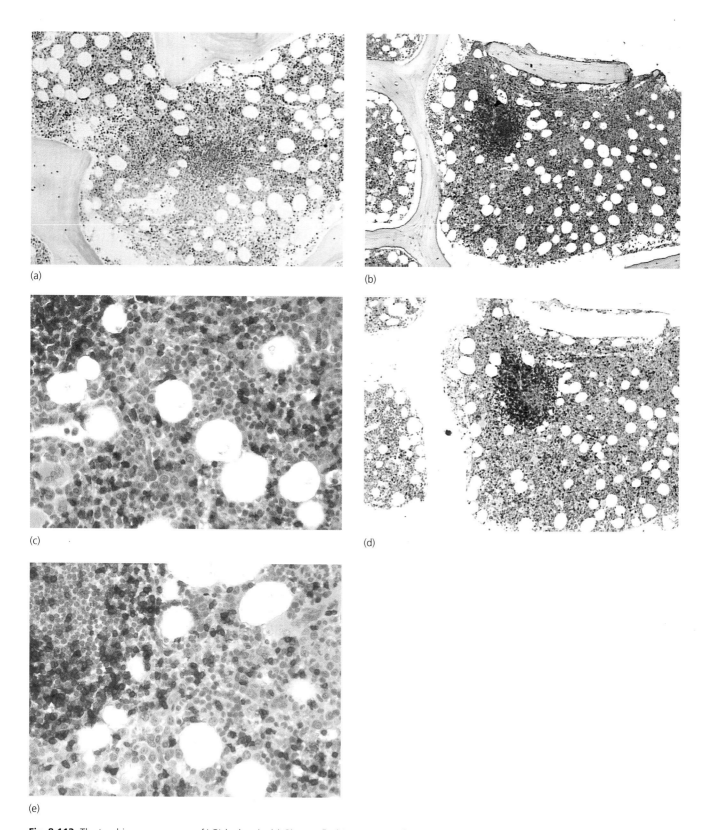

Fig. 8.113 The trephine appearances of LGL leukemia. (a) Giemsa. (b,c) Immunostain for CD20 (B cell). (d,e) Immunostain for CD3.

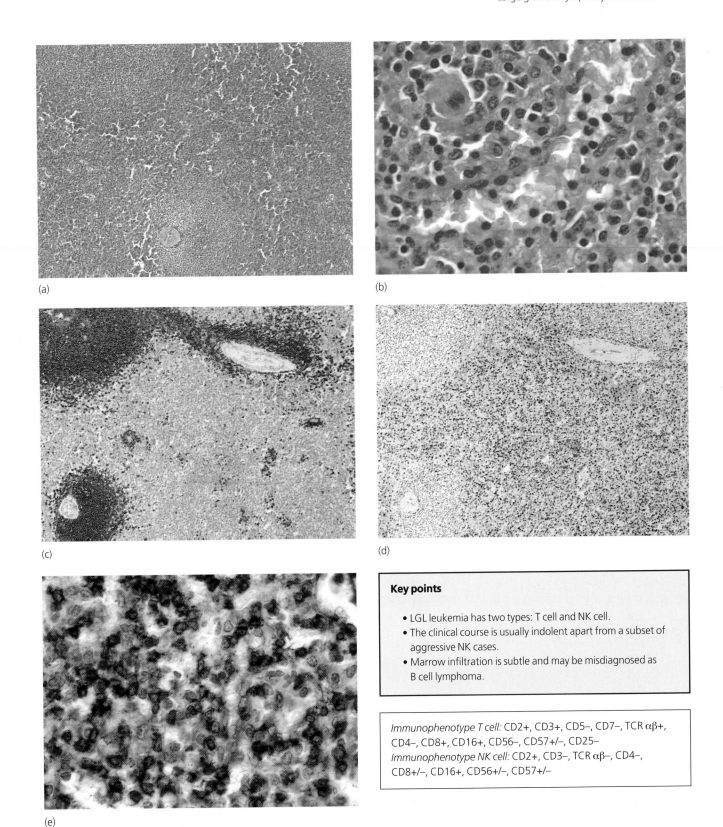

Key points

- LGL leukemia has two types: T cell and NK cell.
- The clinical course is usually indolent apart from a subset of aggressive NK cases.
- Marrow infiltration is subtle and may be misdiagnosed as B cell lymphoma.

Immunophenotype T cell: CD2+, CD3+, CD5–, CD7–, TCR αβ+, CD4–, CD8+, CD16+, CD56–, CD57+/–, CD25–
Immunophenotype NK cell: CD2+, CD3–, TCR αβ–, CD4–, CD8+/–, CD16+, CD56+/–, CD57+/–

Fig. 8.114 The spleen in LGL leukemia. (a,b) H&E. (c) CD20. (d) CD3. (e) CD8.

Chapter 8.13 Cutaneous T cell lymphoma

Most primary lymphomas of the skin are of two T cell types: mycosis fungoides or Sézary syndrome.

Mycosis fungoides more frequently affects middle-aged men and presents with single or multiple scaly skin lesions. The clinical progression is slow, often over 15 or 20 years, and the disease tends to remain localized to the skin although the lesions may become tumorous and ulcerate. Visceral and nodal involvement tends to occur late in the course of the disease.

Sézary syndrome can be viewed as the leukemic counterpart of mycosis fungoides. It also has a cutaneous component but this tends to be much more extensive, existing as a pruritic generalized exfoliating erythroderma ("rouge homme"). Nodal involvement is common. The average life expectancy is 5 years.

Transformation to a large cell lymphoma, often of anaplastic large cell type, may occur as a terminal event in either form of primary cutaneous T cell lymphoma.

Histopathology of the bone marrow

The marrow is rarely involved, even in patients with advanced disease or Sézary syndrome. The neoplastic cell is usually of the T cell helper (CD4) type and morphologically is small with a convoluted (cerebriform) nucleus. Occasional larger cells may be present and these too have convoluted nuclei. There is no characteristic pattern of marrow involvement (Fig. 8.115).

> *Immunophenotype:* CD2+, CD3+, CD5+, CD7+ (30%), CD4+, CD25–

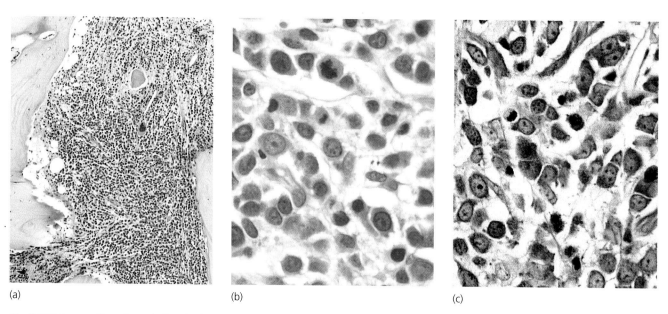

(a) (b) (c)

Fig. 8.115 Large cell lymphoma infiltrating bone marrow as a terminal event in long-standing mycosis fungoides. (a,b) H&E. (c) Giemsa.

Key points

- Primary cutaneous T cell lymphoma has two clinical forms.
- It usually is of T helper immunophenotype.
- The marrow is rarely involved.

Diagnostic problems

The distinctive and readily observed clinical features of this condition and ease with which skin biopsies can be undertaken mean that diagnostic difficulties relating to marrow diagnosis are unlikely.

Chapter 8.14 Peripheral T cell lymphomas, unspecified

The WHO classification recognizes the difficulty faced by histopathologists in subclassifying T cell lymphomas and has included a category called "peripheral T cell lymphoma, unspecified." This category comprises those cases that do not have distinct clinical syndromes that correspond to recognizable morphologic subtypes. While the Kiel classification recognizes as separate entities T zone lymphoma, lymphoepithelioid cell lymphoma (Lennert), T immunoblastic and pleomorphic lymphoma, the WHO classification groups these diseases together under the heading of peripheral T cell lymphoma, unspecified.

The clinical features are varied. Most patients are adults with lymphadenopathy, skin (pruritus) and occasionally abdominal visceral involvement. Eosinophilia and a hemophagocytic syndrome may occur. The clinical course is usually aggressive and histologic grade is less useful as a predictor of clinical behavior than it is for B cell lymphomas.

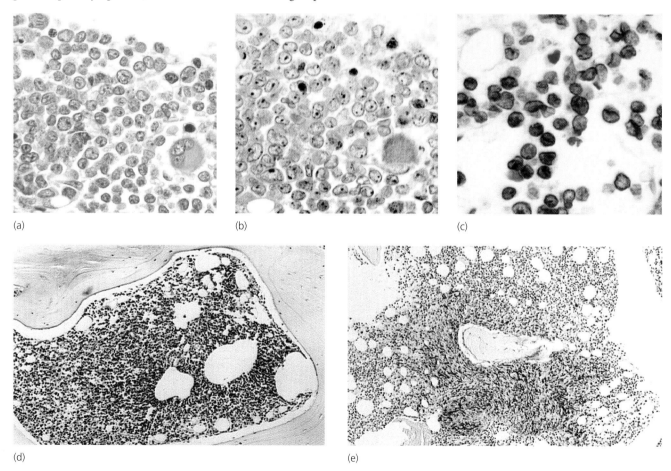

Fig. 8.116 Typical peripheral T cell lymphoma. (a) H&E. (b) Giemsa. (c) Immunostain for CD3. Two different patterns of infiltration are shown by immunostaining for T cells (d,e).

H&E.

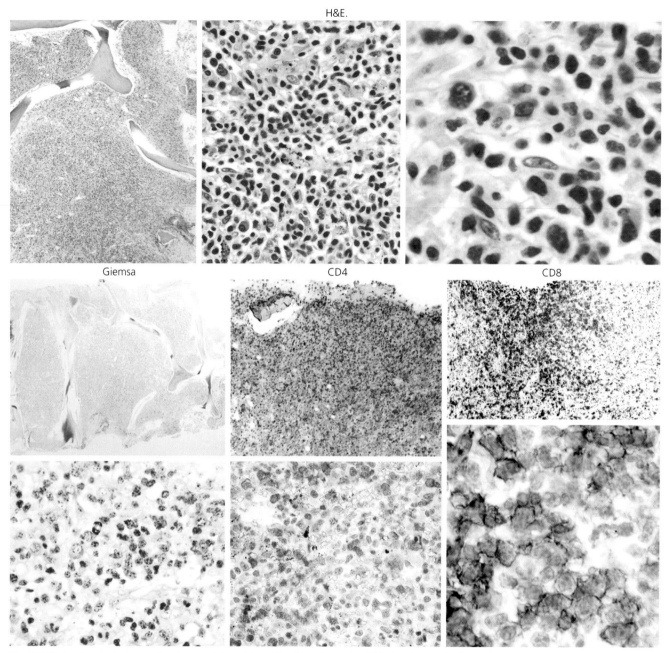

Fig. 8.117 Another typical case of a pleomorphic peripheral T cell lymphoma in which the abnormal cells are CD8 positive but predominantly CD4 negative.

Histopathology of the bone marrow

Given the unspecified nature of this entity it is not surprising that there are no unequivocal figures on marrow involvement. It would appear to be relatively common (i.e. up to 40% of cases). The pattern of infiltration is variable and can be interstitial, paratrabecular or both. The infiltrate is similar to that in the tissues, being polymorphous with variable numbers of small, medium and large neoplastic atypical lymphoid cells admixed with eosinophils and histiocytes, some of which may be epithelioid. The neoplastic cells have irregular nuclei and some larger cells may resemble Reed–Sternberg cells (Fig. 8.116). Although most cases are CD4 positive and CD8 negative, any combination of these two subset markers may occur (Fig. 8.117).

Immunophenotype: CD3+/–, CD2+/–, CD5+/–, CD7–/+,
CD4>CD8 may be CD4–, CD8– may be CD45RA+ and CD45RO–

Key points

- Histologic classification of T cell lymphomas is difficult.
- The WHO classification groups together a number of lymphomas previously recognized as separate entities in other classifications.
- Histologic grading of T cell lymphomas is less predictive of clinical behavior than histologic grading of B cell lymphomas.

Diagnostic problems

In marrows with interstitial involvement it may be difficult to decide whether or not the T cells are truly neoplastic. When only a marrow sample is available for diagnosis it may be impossible to reach a conclusion without parallel molecular investigations.

Chapter 8.15 Hepatosplenic T cell lymphoma

This is a systemic extranodal lymphoma of cytotoxic T cells usually of γδ T cell receptor type. It presents with massive hepatosplenomegaly and the bone marrow is virtually always involved. Patients are generally young adults with profound pancytopenia. The condition is very aggressive, relapses quickly after treatment and has a short median survival of less than 2 years.

Histopathology of the bone marrow

The bone marrow is usually involved although at times it may be difficult to detect the tumor cells even immunocytochemically. The characteristic pattern of involvement is sinusoidal with the rest of the marrow appearing relatively intact (Fig. 8.118).

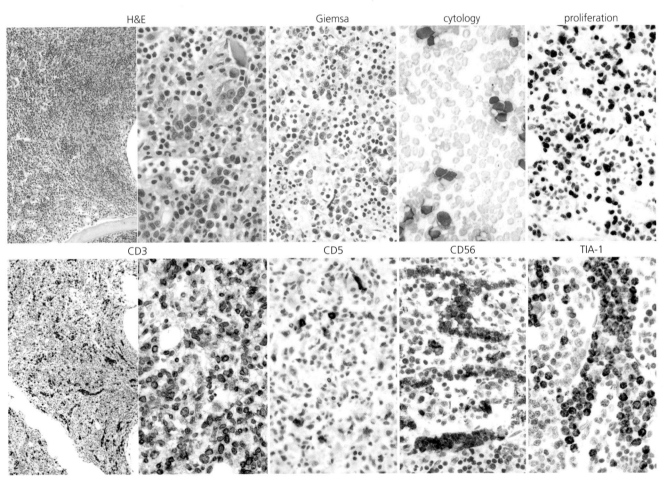

Fig. 8.118 Hepatosplenic T cell lymphoma. On low power examination the infiltrate is subtle but apparent on higher power H&Es or Giemsas as sinusoidal. This pattern is brought out by CD3, CD56 and TIA-1 staining. Note that CD5 is negative: an abnormal T cell phenotype can be useful in identifying a neoplastic T cell population from a reactive one.

Diagnostic problems

Because this lymphoma is extranodal, a bone marrow biopsy may be the preliminary diagnostic specimen. Unless a diagnosis of lymphoma was expected clinically, it can be easy to overlook the infiltration unless immunostaining is requested. Conditions such as this are examples of the value of performing a simple B and T cell screen on any marrow where the diagnosis is clinically unclear. Once the sinusoidal T cells are spotted, a fuller immunophenotype may be completed and a diagnosis reached.

Immunophenotype: CD2+, CD3+, CD5−, CD7−, TCR δ1+, CD4−, CD8−, CD16+, CD56+, TIA-1+

Key point

- Bone marrow usually involved at diagnosis but may be difficult to detect without immunostaining.

Chapter 8.16 Angioimmunoblastic T cell lymphoma

This is an uncommon condition that is clinically distinct and has a variable clinical course with occasional remissions and relapses, but often transforming into a frank high-grade lymphoma (mostly T cell but occasionally secondary EBV positive B cell lymphoma). Patients usually have fever, generalized lymphadenopathy, skin rash and raised polyclonal gammaglobulins.

Histopathology of the bone marrow

The diagnosis of angioimmunoblastic lymphoma requires a lymph node biopsy (Fig. 8.119). The marrow is involved in a significant number of cases (Fig. 8.120). Focal areas of fibrosis and increased vascularization are seen although the complex arborizing vasculature with periodic acid–Schiff (PAS) positive walls seen in affected lymph nodes is much less obvious and may be absent. Within these areas, a highly polymorphic cell population is found. Reactive and neoplastic cells are intimately admixed and include plasma cells, eosinophils, epithelioid macrophages together with the neoplastic small- and medium-sized lymphocytes and immunoblasts.

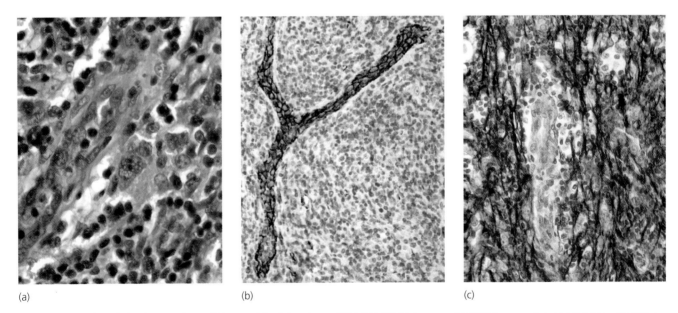

(a)　　　　　　　　　(b)　　　　　　　　　(c)

Fig. 8.119 Lymph node involvement by angioimmunoblastic lymphoma (AIL). (a) H&E, high power. (b) CD31 immunostain highlighting vascularity. (c) CD21 immunostain showing dendritic reticulin cell meshwork around vessels.

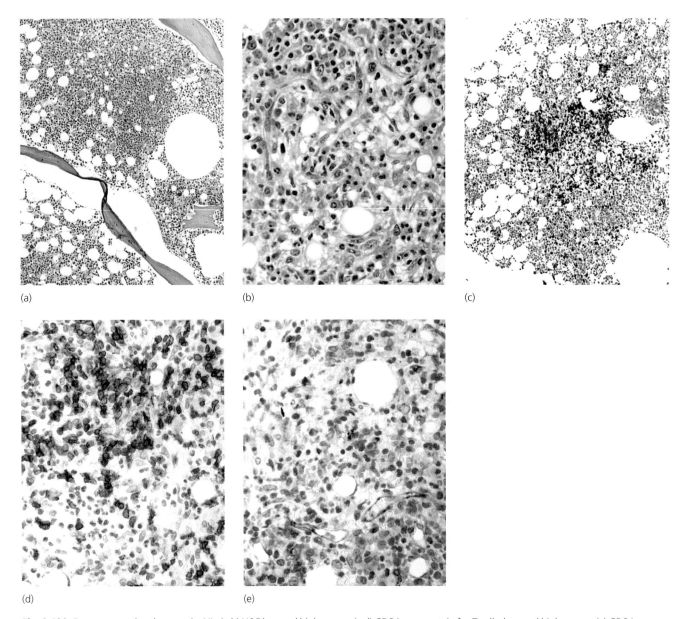

Fig. 8.120 Bone marrow involvement in AIL. (a,b) H&E low and high power. (c,d) CD3 immunostain for T cells, low and high power. (e) CD31 immunostain for endothelial cells.

The immunophenotypic pattern is characteristic. The abnormal cells have a full T cell phenotype and are mainly of CD4 subtype. These T cells also typically express CD10 in lymph nodes although this can be difficult to detect in the bone marrow (perhaps somewhat similarly to the situation with follicular lymphoma; see Fig 8.59).

Immunophenotype: CD2+, CD3+, CD4+/–, CD5+, CD7+, CD8–, CD10–/+

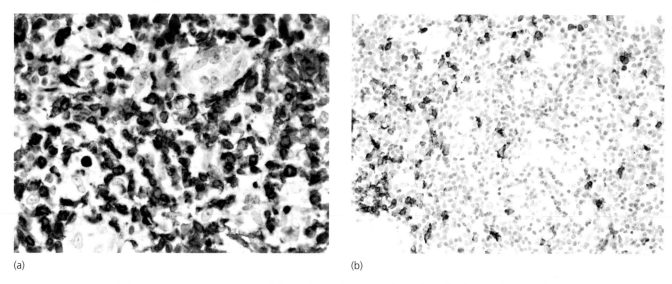

(a)   (b)

Fig. 8.121 Case of AIL in the bone marrow where although the majority of the infiltrating cells are T cells (CD3+) a surprising number are medium-to large-sized B cells (CD20). Many of the B cells will express Epstein–Barr virus (EBV) antigens.

Diagnostic problems

Angioimmunoblastic lymphoma vs. Hodgkin lymphoma

The fibrosis, focal nature of the disease within the marrow and the mixed inflammatory cell infiltrate including eosinophils might indicate a diagnosis of Hodgkin lymphoma. The distinction will best be made on the lymph node biopsy although immunostaining will be helpful if no other material is available. In angioimmunoblastic lymphoma (AIL) the abnormal large cells are usually T cells (but occasionally B cells) with little expression of CD30 and no CD15 positivity (Fig 8.121).

Key points

- Angioimmunoblastic lymphoma has a variable clinical course.
- Marrow lesions lack the characteristic architectural features seen in lymph nodes.
- Differential diagnosis includes Hodgkin lymphoma and mastocytosis.

Angioimmunoblastic lymphoma vs. mastocytosis

Mastocytosis may also involve the marrow in a similar way and a mixed inflammatory infiltrate is not uncommon. The fibrosis and increased number of endothelial cells may produce an appearance of a spindled cell population in AIL similar to the spindled mast cells in mastocytosis. The mast cell granules are likely to be identified in most instances of mastocytosis on Giemsa stain. Immunostaining for T cell (CD3), macrophage markers (CD68), mast cell tryptase and c-kit (CD117) (the latter three being positive in mastocytosis) will also be helpful.

Chapter 8.17 Adult T cell lymphoma/leukemia

This is a rare condition in the West and was originally described in patients from Japan and later the Caribbean. It is caused by the human T cell lymphotropic virus (HTLV-1), a type C retrovirus. It usually involves adults and has an aggressive course with leukemia, hypercalcemia, hepatosplenomegaly and lytic bone lesions. Rare cases with an indolent clinical course and mild lymphocytosis have been described. Patients have antibodies to HTLV-1. Characteristic clover-leaf lymphocytes are seen in the peripheral blood.

Histopathology of the bone marrow

The marrow is involved in the majority of cases and tends to have a diffuse pattern which ranges from sparse to packed. There is marked cellular pleomorphism and the variation in cell size from case to case is great (Fig. 8.122).

Large cells may resemble Reed–Sternberg cells. Mitotic figures are easily found. Increased osteoclast activity with bone resorption may be seen, even in the absence of a demonstrable lymphoma infiltrate (Fig. 8.122).

Reactive features include increased vascularization, eosinophils and plasma cells.

Diagnostic problems

Serologic investigation for HTLV antibodies in suspected cases will confirm or refute the diagnosis. On histologic grounds alone it may not be possible to distinguish adult T cell lymphoma involvement of the marrow from other T cell lymphoma infiltrates. The presence of Reed–Sternberg-like cells in some cases should not lead to a misdiagnosis of Hodgkin lymphoma because the associated neoplastic infiltrate of small- and medium-sized pleomorphic cells would not be a feature of Hodgkin lymphoma. In cases where there is still doubt the clinical picture of a leukemia will readily make the distinction.

Rare cases of adult T cell lymphoma without leukemia have been reported and this possibility should be borne in mind in cases with an atypical clinical presentation.

> *Immunophenotype:* CD2+, CD3+, CD4+, CD5+, CD25+, CD7–, CD8–

Key points

- Adult T cell lymphoma is caused by a retrovirus, HTLV-1.
- The disease is usually clinically aggressive.
- The marrow is involved to varying degrees in the majority of patients.
- The neoplastic cells tend to be highly pleomorphic.
- Patients will have antibodies to HTLV-1.

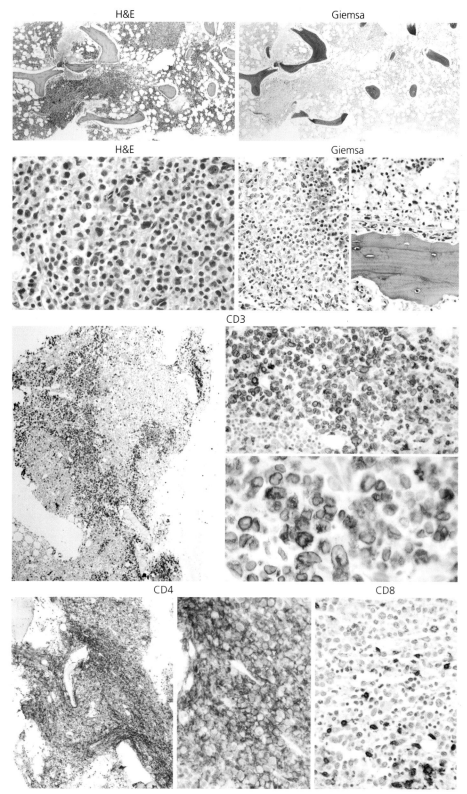

Fig. 8.122 The marrow may be patchily (as shown here) or diffusely infiltrated by pleomorphic cells as shown at higher power in the second row. Typically, increased osteoblastic and osteoclastic activity is present as seen in the second higher power (Giemsa). The abnormal cells are usually positive for CD2, CD3, CD4 and CD5 but lack CD7 or CD8.

Chapter 8.18 Anaplastic large cell lymphoma

This is a T cell lymphoma generally composed of large and somewhat cohesive cells whose identity was revealed by antibody Ki-1[1] recognizing the key presence of CD30 in these lymphomas. Many cases stain for one or more T cell antigens with CD43 being the most frequent (although of course this is not lineage specific). The tumor cells may lack all of the regular T cell antigens used in diagnosis and are then often referred to as "null" cell cases. However, most of these still have T cell gene rearrangements indicating their underlying T cell lineage. The majority of cases are positive for anaplastic large cell lymphoma kinase (ALK) protein because of chromosomal translocations involving the *alk* gene on chromosome 2.[2] The most common translocation is t(2;5), which causes nuclear and cytoplasmic localization of ALK (Fig. 8.123).

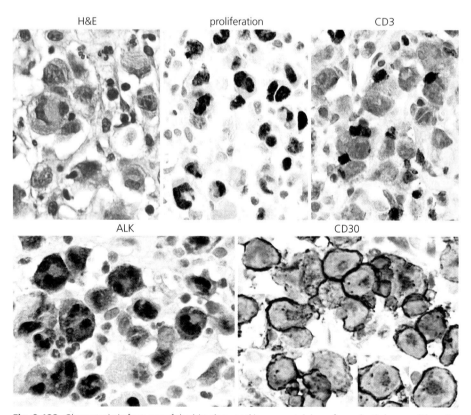

Fig. 8.123 Characteristic features of the histology and immunostaining of anaplastic large cell lymphoma (ALCL). The proliferation is high in the large cohesive anaplastic tumor cells. The T cell antigen CD3 is often weak and cytoplasmic and anaplastic large cell lymphoma kinase (ALK) is both nuclear and cytoplasmic. CD30 is always positive (almost by definition).

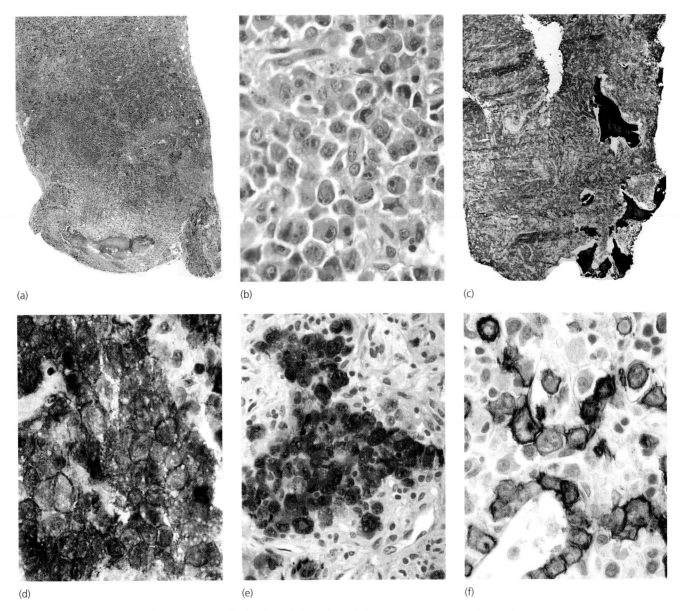

Fig. 8.124 Bone marrow involvement by ALCL. (a,b) H&E. (c,d) CD30. (e) ALK. (f) Epithelial membrane antigen (EMA).

Anaplastic large cell lymphoma (ALCL) may involve lymph nodes or extranodal sites (e.g. soft tissue, bone and skin) and behaves in a clinically aggressive manner similar to the other large cell lymphomas. It usually arises *de novo* but a few cases have occurred in patients with pre-existing Hodgkin lymphoma. It has a bimodal age distribution (i.e. older children and the elderly) and may possibly have a better prognosis in children than other childhood high-grade large cell lymphomas.

Initially it was believed that ALCL could include B cell cases but because these lack the translocations with chromosome 2 seen in most of the T cell cases they are now classified with the diffuse large B cell lymphomas. In addition, it was initially thought that ALCL had two clinical forms: the systemic and the cutaneous. However, the latter is now seen as a separate entity and is classified as a primary cutaneous CD30-positive T cell lymphoproliferative disorder.[3] It has a much better prognosis than ALCL.

Although ALCL has only recently been characterized as an entity, it is not a new disease and has probably been misdiagnosed as a number of different conditions in the past, such as metastatic carcinoma, amelanotic melanoma, lymphocyte-depleted Hodgkin lymphoma, malignant histiocytosis, sarcoma and regressing atypical histiocytosis.

Histopathology of the bone marrow

The neoplastic cells have a distinctive morphology. They are large, have abundant cytoplasm and large pleomorphic kidney-shaped nuclei with prominent multiple eosinophilic nucleoli. The irregular nuclear contours have led to varied fanciful descriptions such as "jellyfish," "embryo" and "foot-print" like. The cells appear to adhere to each other, resulting in a cohesive growth pattern. Large sheets of cells often occur and impart a syncytial appearance. Mitotic figures are easily seen. Marrow involvement is rarely subtle and a focal or diffuse pattern is seen. The diagnosis rests on the immunohisto-chemistry (Fig. 8.124).

Diagnostic problems

The cohesive growth pattern of this lymphoma means that it is often mistaken morphologically for metastatic carcinoma. In addition, the positivity for epithelial membrane antigen (EMA), and negativity for leukocyte common antigen (CD45) in most cases, enlarge this diagnostic trap. A wider panel of antibodies, to include anti-cytokeratins and CD30, normally permits a distinction between these two conditions. Anti-melanoma markers (e.g. S-100 and HMB45) should also be included.

Some cases may show morphologic similarities with Hodgkin lymphoma. However, because ALCL is a T cell neoplasm and Hodgkin lymphoma is largely a B-cell-derived neoplasm, immunohistochemistry (for CD15, pan-B and pan-T, EMA and ALK) and antigen-receptor gene rearrange-ment studies (albeit very difficult to perform in most cases of Hodgkin lymphoma) usually permit a distinction to be made. The WHO classification (unlike the REAL classification) there-fore does not recognize a Hodgkin-related ALCL category.

Immunophenotype: CD30+, EMA+/−, ALK+/−, CD45−/+, CD25+/−, CD15−/+, CD2 & CD4+/−, CD3, CD5 & CD7 −/+, CD43+/−

Key points

- ALCL has a characteristic morphology and immunophenotype.
- ALCL has two clinical forms: systemic and primary cutaneous.
- Its cohesive growth pattern may mimic metastatic carcinoma.
- An unclear relationship between ALCL and Hodgkin lymphoma exists.

References

1 Stein H, Mason D, Gerdes J, *et al.* The expression of the Hodgkin's disease associated antigen Ki-1 in reactive and neoplastic lymphoid tissue: evidence that Reed–Sternberg cells and histiocytic malignan-cies are derived from activated lymphoid cells. *Blood* 1985; **66**: 848–58.

2 Benharroch D, Meguerian-Bedoyan Z, Lamant L, *et al.* ALK-positive lymphoma: a single disease with a broad spectrum of morphology. *Blood* 1998; **91**: 2076–84.

3 Beljaards RC, Kaudewitz P, Berti E, *et al.* Primary cutaneous CD30-positive large cell lymphoma: definition of a new type of cutaneous lymphoma with a favorable prognosis. A European Multicenter Study of 47 patients. *Cancer* 1993; **71**: 2097–104.

Chapter 9 Hodgkin lymphoma

Hodgkin lymphoma is a lymphoma characterized by the presence of large binucleate Reed–Sternberg (RS) cells in a background of reactive-appearing lymphocytes, macrophages, granulocytes and fibroblasts. Its exact etiology is unknown. The neoplastic cells are now believed to be derived from germinal center B cells in most (>98%) cases. They possess unique non-coding mutations in their rearranged immunoglobulin genes accounting for the lack of traditional B cell properties and hence the time it took to establish their lineage. In the light of these findings the WHO authors decided that Hodgkin's disease should be relabeled Hodgkin lymphoma. This has not met with universal approval and we have stated elsewhere it is probably sensible if pathologists and clinicians adopt whichever term they feel gives them best usage. For example, if we still believe it is valuable clinically to distinguish Hodgkin's from non-Hodgkin's then one could argue that keeping the term Hodgkin's disease reduces confusion or misunderstanding. To avoid confusion in this text we have used the WHO term Hodgkin lymphoma throughout.

The WHO classification divides Hodgkin lymphoma into lymphocyte predominant and classic varieties (mixed cellularity, nodular sclerosing, lymphocyte depleted and lymphocyte rich). It is now clear that lymphocyte-predominant is a separate entity and is a form of B cell follicular proliferation with a predisposition (3–5% of cases) to develop into a large B cell lymphoma.

The classic varieties are almost the same as those categorized in the 1966 RYE classification apart from the addition of a lymphocyte rich variant. Lymphocyte depleted has become an uncommon diagnosis, with most cases being reclassified as anaplastic large cell lymphomas.

Clinical features

Hodgkin lymphoma usually presents with painless enlargement of one or more groups of lymph nodes. A history of lymph node enlargement for several weeks or months is not uncommon. The affected lymph nodes may already be quite large when first noticed, and subsequent growth may often be negligible or the nodes may shrink or fluctuate in size. The enlarged lymph nodes are firm, non-tender and often feel rubbery. Non-specific hematologic abnormalities are common but bone marrow involvement at presentation is uncommon (especially now that so many cases previously diagnosed as lymphocyte depleted have been reclassified as non-Hodgkin lymphomas). Hodgkin lymphoma in the bone marrow is more frequent at relapse. Usually, the abnormal cells do not smear out onto the aspirate so that histology is vital in making the diagnosis. Rarely, Hodgkin cells may spill out into the peripheral blood (Fig. 9.1).

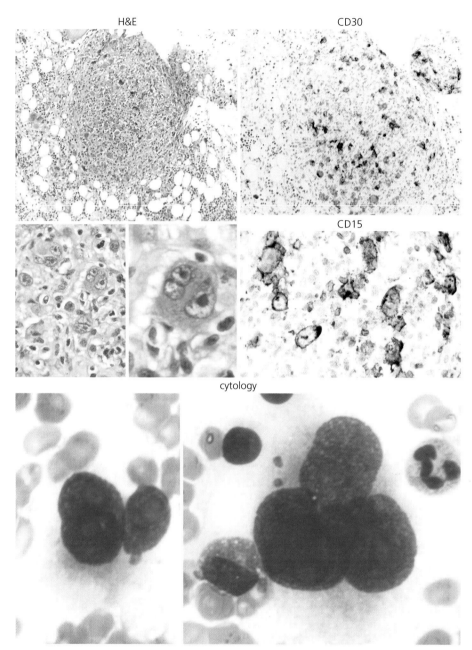

Fig. 9.1 Unusual case of classic Hodgkin lymphoma in which the abnormal cells appeared in both the peripheral blood (lower left) and in the bone marrow aspirate (lower right). The lymph node features are shown in the two upper rows.

Histopathology of the bone marrow

Classic Hodgkin lymphoma

The bone marrow appearances of mixed cellularity or nodular sclerosis are indistinguishable so that subtyping must be performed on a lymph node biopsy. Usually, the marrow shows focal involvement emphasizing the importance of an adequate-sized trephine specimen when staging Hodgkin lymphoma. In most cases of nodal disease with spread to the marrow, diagnostic cells are rare (Fig. 9.2) but a combination of focal fibrosis and abnormal mononuclear cells (RS cells are not essential if node involvement has been confirmed histologically) with appropriate immunostaining will allow a confident diagnosis (Fig. 9.3).

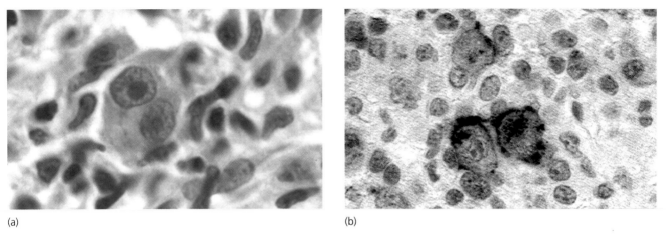

(a)

(b)

Fig. 9.2 Diagnostic Reed–Sternberg cell in the bone marrow. (a) H&E. (b) Immunostain for CD30.

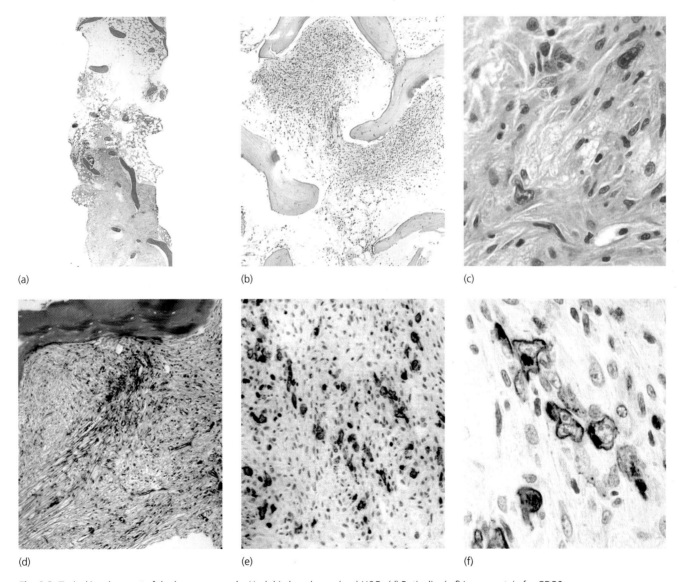

(a)

(b)

(c)

(d)

(e)

(f)

Fig. 9.3 Typical involvement of the bone marrow by Hodgkin lymphoma (a–c) H&E. (d) Reticulin. (e,f) Immunostain for CD30.

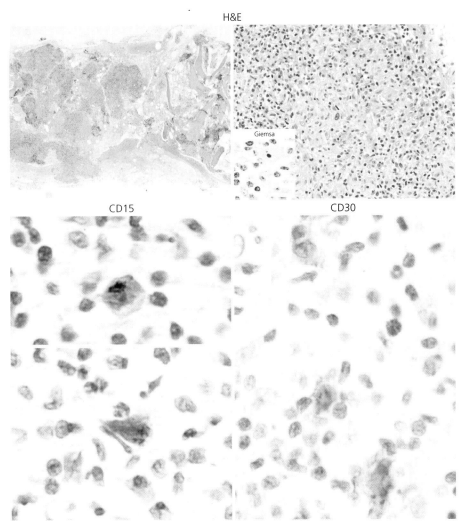

Fig. 9.4 Case of a child who presented with pancytopenia but no other signs. A bone marrow biopsy shown here revealed Hodgkin lymphoma. Treatment (after exhaustive clinical discussion) was initially successful but after some months the child relapsed with widespread classic Hodgkin lymphoma to which he subsequently succumbed.

It is frequently useful to include antibodies recognizing megakaryocytes to be certain that the abnormal cells are truly derived from Hodgkin lymphoma. It is very unusual for Hodgkin lymphoma of any subtype to present solely as a bone marrow infiltration. In such cases it will be essential to identify a definite RS cell (Fig. 9.4).

The characteristic immunophenotype of Hodgkin lymphoma is CD30 and CD15 positive. This is diagnostic as no other tumor known to us has this combination of markers. Unfortunately, CD15 is not expressed by all cases, being positive in approximately 75% of cases. In many cases, one needs a careful examination of the sections to find CD15 positive cells as they may be in a minority and demonstrate only a dot-like staining pattern. This is fine in lymph nodes but very difficult in the bone marrow where CD15 is a strong marker of myeloid cells and assessing whether or not a single large cell is positive and abnormal can be perilous (Fig. 9.5). The B cell markers PAX5 and MUM1 can be helpful in this situation in association with negativity for CD20.

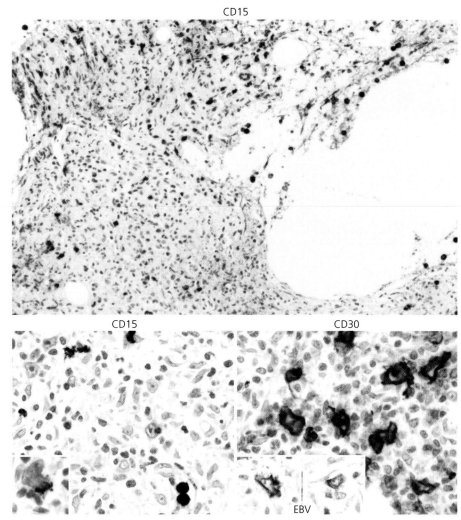

Fig. 9.5 This case illustrates CD15 positivity in a case of classical Hodgkin lymphoma. Note that CD15 also stains strongly granulocytes shown in the top picture at the right. CD15 is also positive on only a minority of the Hodgkin cells as compared with CD30 (bottom right). Epstein–Barr virus (EBV) can also occasionally be detected in Hodgkin lymphoma in the bone marrow (bottom right insert).

Nodular lymphocyte predominant Hodgkin lymphoma

Since the recognition of this condition as a separate entity it is clear that bone marrow involvement is rare, other than when there has been a transformation to a large B cell lymphoma (Fig. 9.6).

Immunophenotype classic Reed–Sternberg cells:
    CD15+, CD30+, CD45-, EMA–/+, J chain–
    PAX5+, MUM1+, CD20–/+
    BOB1–, Oct2–/+
    Other B cell antigens rare
Immunophenotype lymphocyte predominant (L&H) cells:
    CD15–, CD30–, CD45+, EMA+/–, J chain+
    PAX5+, MUM1–, CD20+
    BOB.1+, Oct2+,
    CD10–, bcl6+
    Other B cell antigens +

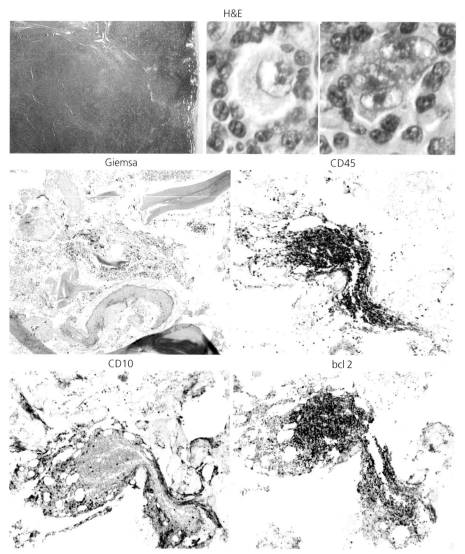

H&E

Giemsa   CD45

CD10   bcl 2

Fig. 9.6 Nodular lymphocyte predominant Hodgkin lymphoma involving the bone marrow. The typical lymph node appearances are shown in the top row. The marrow (bottom two rows) was rather crushed but there was a clear-cut paratrabecular aggregate better seen in the immunostains than in the Giemsa.

Diagnostic problems

Other fibrosing conditions

Superficially the abnormal cells in fibrosing myeloproliferative conditions and secondary carcinoma can look like Hodgkin cells. The key to avoiding these errors is not to diagnose Hodgkin lymphoma on a marrow alone without careful clinical review of the case. Appropriate immunostaining for megakaryocytes and epithelial cells should be undertaken in addition to that for Hodgkin lymphoma (Fig. 9.7).

The distinction from anaplastic large cell lymphoma (ALCL) can also be troublesome. Again a careful immunophenotype, especially looking for B cell antigens (Hodgkin) and ALK (ALCL), will greatly assist.

Hodgkin lymphoma in the bone marrow can also be associated with profound granulomatous reactions that can easily mask the underlying malignancy (Fig. 9.8). Remember to perform appropriate granuloma stains such as a Ziehl–Neelsen (ZN) because other causes such as tuberculosis (TB) may coexist with Hodgkin lymphoma especially if human immunodeficiency virus (HIV) is implicated.

H&E

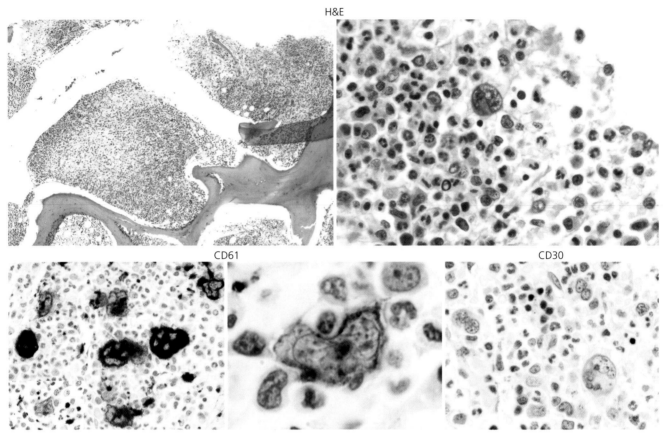

CD61   CD30

Fig. 9.7 Bone marrow from a patient with a myeloproliferative disorder where the abnormal megakaryocytes raised the possibility of Hodgkin lymphoma. Immunostains for CD61 and CD30 identified their true character.

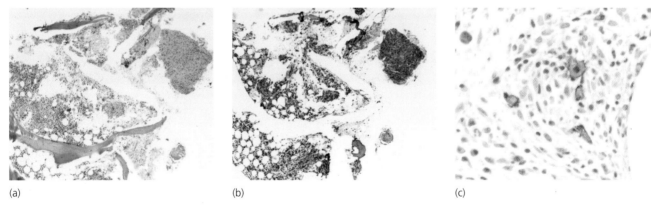

(a)   (b)   (c)

Fig. 9.8 Extensive granuloma formation in the bone marrow shown by (a) H&E and (b) CD68 (macrophage) staining. The underlying Hodgkin lymphoma can only clearly be seen on (c) CD30 immunostaining. A Ziehl–Neelsen (ZN) stain was negative.

Key points

- Classic Hodgkin lymphoma causes a fibrotic response, typically patchy in the bone marrow.
- Involvement of the marrow is rare at presentation but relatively common at relapse.
- Immunocytochemical examination is helpful in distinguishing it from other fibrosing conditions of the bone marrow and from anaplastic large cell lymphoma.

Chapter 10 Metastatic disease

Metastatic spread of carcinoma and sarcoma to the bone marrow is relatively common as a terminal event when there is usually little or no clinical justification for a biopsy. In practice, the number of trephines taken for diagnosis of secondary disease, including those discovered by chance, is small. In our own practice, the last 9000 bone marrow trephines contained just over 100 diagnoses of metastatic disease, which is only a little over 1% of cases.

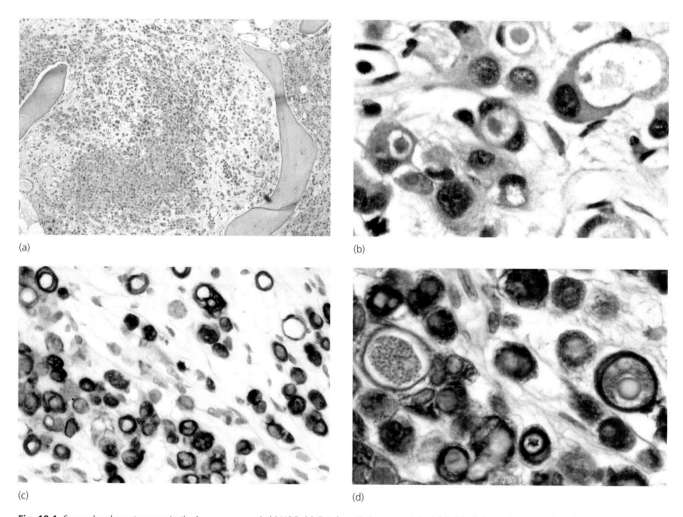

(a) (b) (c) (d)

Fig. 10.1 Secondary breast cancer in the bone marrow. (a,b) H&E. (c) Cytokeratin immunostain. (d) Epithelial membrane antigen (EMA) immunostain.

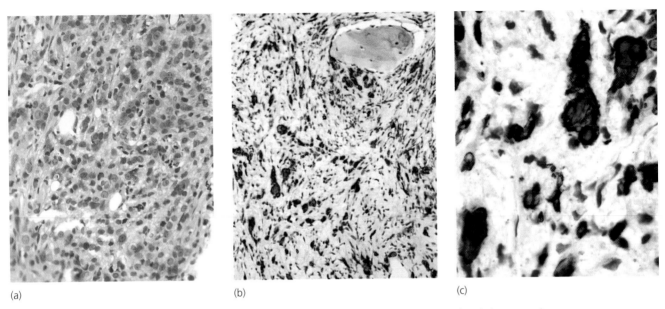

Fig. 10.2 Extensive fibrosis in the marrow from secondary cancer of unknown origin. (a) H&E. (b,c) Cytokeratin immunostain.

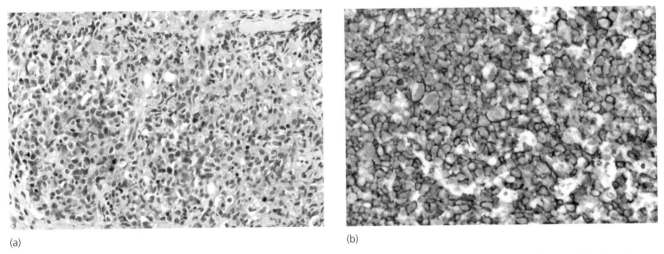

Fig. 10.3 Secondary tumor that was confidently diagnosed as a carcinoma until a review was prompted by clinical doubts. It was a diffuse large B cell lymphoma as revealed by CD20 immunostaining. (a) H&E, (b) CD20.

Clinical features

Except in pediatric diseases, staging biopsies are rarely taken in the UK. Most biopsies are for unexplained anemias or localized bone pain when a diagnosis of myeloma is part of the differential. Often, a leukoerythroblastic blood picture (characterized by circulating immature granulocytes, nucleated red cells, abnormal platelets and teardrop erythrocytes) is also present.

Histopathology of the bone marrow

Carcinoma

The bone marrow is virtually always grossly abnormal even at low power. Either the marrow will be heavily infiltrated by recognizable tumor (Fig. 10.1) or extensively fibrosed (Fig. 10.2). In both cases immunocytochemistry is useful to ensure that lymphoma is not overlooked (Fig. 10.3). Occasionally, the site of the primary tumor is unclear clinically so that immunostaining for endocrine and prostatic antigens can be helpful (Figs 10.4 and 10.5).

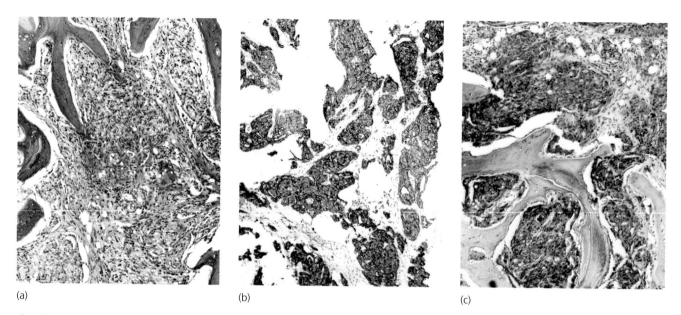

(a) (b) (c)

Fig. 10.4 Extensive prostatic cancer in the bone marrow. (a) Giemsa. (b) Cytokeratin immunostain. (c) Immunostain for prostate-specific antigen.

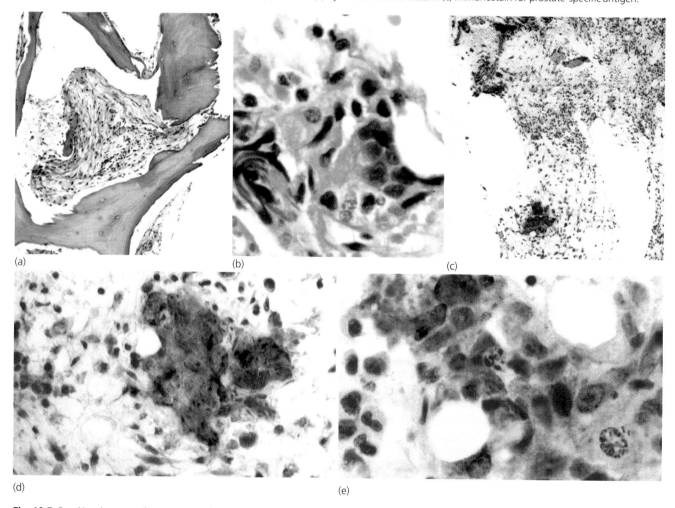

(a) (b) (c)

(d) (e)

Fig. 10.5 Focal involvement of bone marrow by prostatic cancer. (a,b) H&E, note bony sclerosis. (c,d) Immunostain for cytokeratin. (e) Immunostain for prostate-specific antigen.

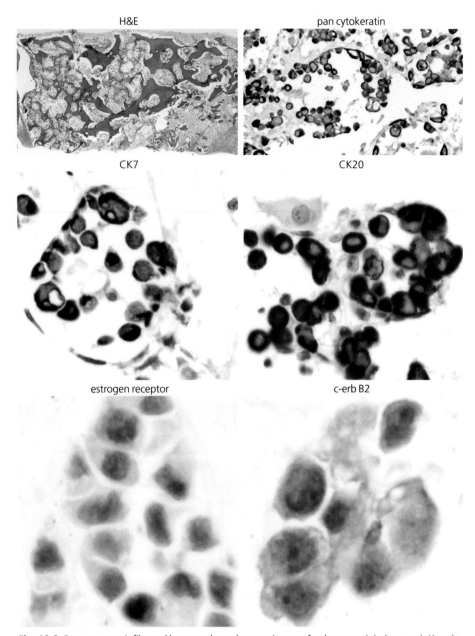

Fig. 10.6 Bone marrow infiltrated by secondary adenocarcinoma of unknown origin (top row). Keratin subtyping (middle row) showed this to be positive for both CK7 and CK20 so that the tumor was eventually traced to the pancreas. A different case was identified as a relapse of a previous breast cancer by staining for estrogen receptor and c-erb B2 (bottom row).

More recently, cytokeratin subtyping has been found to be of some value in tracing the primary site of a tumor[1] while further work on breast cancer has identified markers of value for that site too (Fig. 10.6).

Several studies have shown that multiple biopsies taken at first presentation with a tumor such as breast cancer will demonstrate micrometastases in a proportion of cases. The relevance of these findings to clinical practice or prognosis remains unclear.

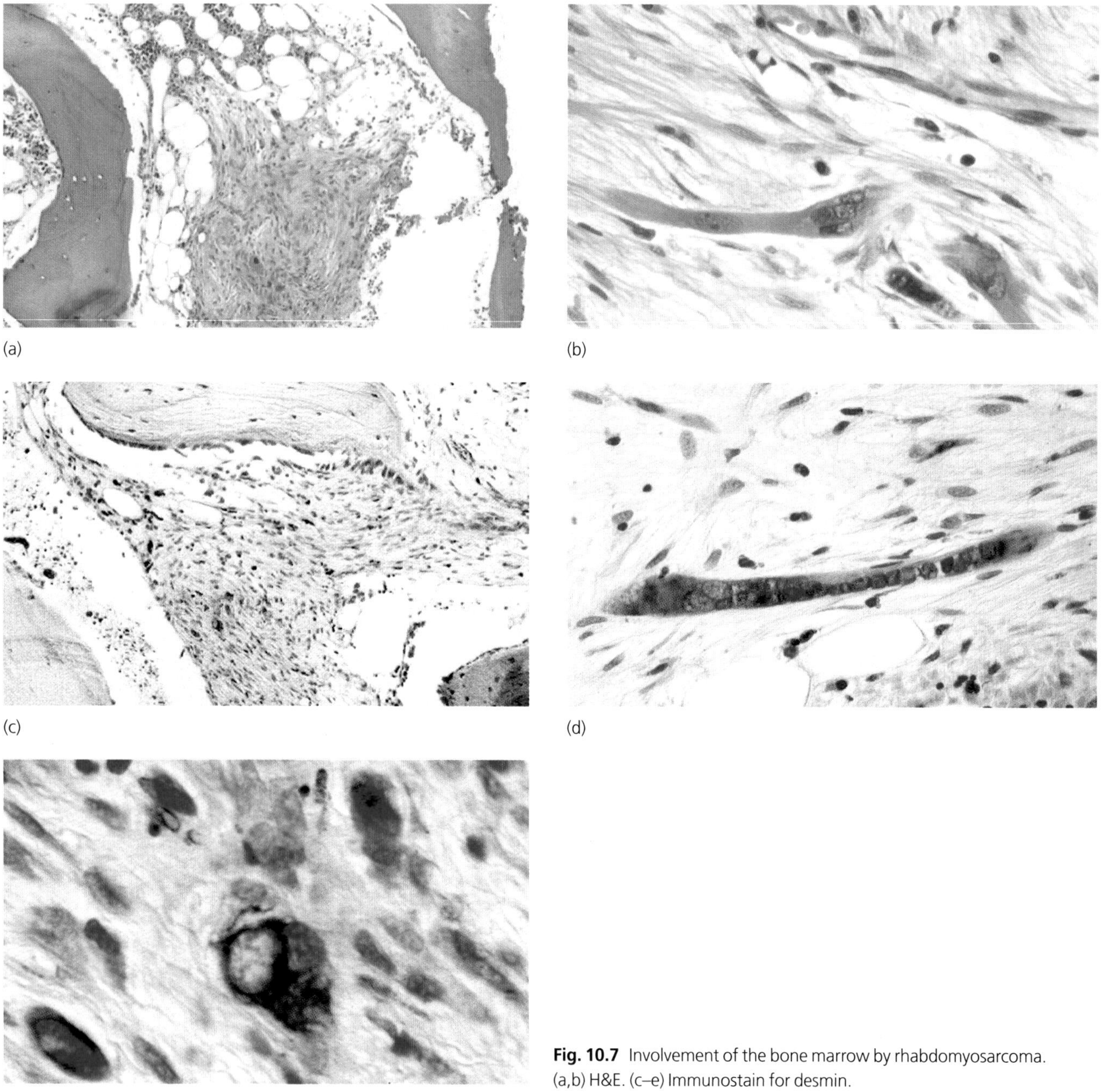

(a)

(b)

(c)

(d)

(e)

Fig. 10.7 Involvement of the bone marrow by rhabdomyosarcoma. (a,b) H&E. (c–e) Immunostain for desmin.

Pediatric tumors

Bone marrow trephines are taken as part of most oncology protocols for the assessment of solid tumors in childhood. Children with disseminated disease are usually identified by the clinician so marrow involvement is rarely a surprise. The differential diagnosis mainly involves neuroblastoma (and its variants), rhabdomyosarcoma and Ewing tumor. It is very uncommon to find such tumors unexpectedly but if this arises a small panel of antibodies aimed at the "small round blue cell tumors of childhood" will usually help to point one in the right direction (Figs 10.7 and 10.8). The differential diagnosis of pediatric tumors is becoming a specialist (and rather complicated) subject in its own right and it is beyond the scope of the current authors to delineate it further without becoming dangerously misleading to readers. Some general pointers are given in Tables 10.1 and 10.2 but it is becoming clear that overlap is greater than previously thought for many of these (e.g. CD99 is present in acute lymphoblastic leukemia as well as in Ewing tumor).

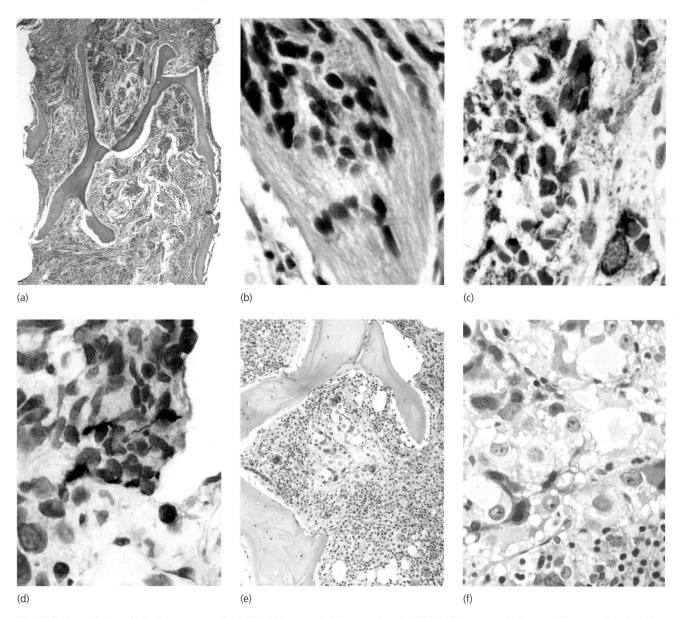

Fig. 10.8 Neuroblastoma in the bone marrow. (a,b) H&E. (c) Immunostain for neural marker NB84. (d) Immunostain for neurofilaments. Occasionally, neuroblastoma may be present in a differentiated form as ganglioneuroblastoma. (e,f) H&E.

Diagnostic problems

Other fibrosing conditions

It is important not to diagnose any fibrotic marrow in a patient with a known history of carcinoma as having metastatic disease without supporting proof such as clear-cut tumor in the marrow or immunocytochemical identification of infiltrating cells. Patients with carcinoma can and do get other diseases such as myelofibrosis.

Key points

- Metastatic disease is a relatively uncommon indication for a bone marrow trephine.
- Involvement of the marrow is usually obvious.
- Immunocytochemical examination is helpful in distinguishing it from other fibrosing conditions of the bone marrow and in identifying different types of tumor.

Reference

1   Chu PG, Weiss LM. Keratin expression in human tissues and neoplasms. *Histopathology* 2002; **40**: 403–39.

Table 10.1 Immunocytochemical identification of carcinomas and pediatric tumors.

Carcinoma

Generic
Cytokeratin+, epithelial membrane antigen (EMA)+, CD45–
Keratin subtyping (see Table 10.2)

Thyroid
Thyroglobulin+, calcitonin+ (medullary)
TTF-1+

Prostate
Prostatic acid phosphatase or prostate-specific antigen+

Breast
Estrogen receptor+, progesteron receptor+
c-Erb B2+

Pediatric tumors

Neuroblastoma
NB84+, neurofilaments+, NCam+

Rhabdomyosarcoma
Desmin+, myoglobin+, WT1+, myogenin+

Ewing tumor
NB84+, neurofilaments-, NCam-, CD99+ (mic2), CD117+ (c-kit)

Table 10.2 Patterns of expression of keratins CK7 and CK20 in epithelial malignancies.

CK7+ CK20+	CK7+ CK20–	CK7– CK20–	CK7– CK20+
Transitional cell	Breast	Hepatocellular renal cell	Colorectal
Pancreatic	Non-small cell lung	Prostate	
Ovarian mucinous	Ovarian serous	Squamous neuroendocrine	
Merkel cell	Mesothelioma		
	Endometrial pancreatic		

Chapter 11 Miscellaneous

This chapter brings together those conditions that do not warrant chapters of their own.

Amyloidosis

This is a rare finding in a marrow biopsy. The amount of amyloid present is variable and the histologic changes may be subtle, requiring a high index of suspicion for its detection. It is present in the walls of vessels and also within the stroma surrounding the hematopoietic tissue. As in other tissues it is extracellular and can be demonstrated histochemically using the Congo red stain. This stains the amyloid orange and displays a brilliant light green color under polarized light (Fig. 11.1). In marrows containing amyloid derived from immunoglobulin light chain, a neoplastic clone of plasma cells may also be detected.

Immune thrombocytopenic purpura

Immune thrombocytopenic purpura (ITP) is caused by the removal of antibody-coated platelets from the circulation. The auto-antibodies are produced by the body in a number of different circumstances, the most common being:

1 autoimmune disorders (e.g. systemic lupus erythematosus [SLE]);
2 viral infections (e.g. human immunodeficiency virus [HIV], Epstein–Barr virus [EBV], cytomegalovirus [CMV]);
3 drug induced (e.g. carbamazepine, chlorothiazide);
4 lymphoproliferative disorders (e.g. Hodgkin's disease [Hodgkin lymphoma], chronic lymphocytic leukemia [CLL]);
5 idiopathic (i.e. of unknown origin).

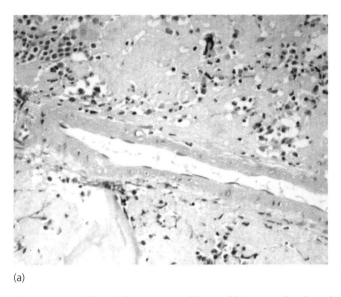
(a)

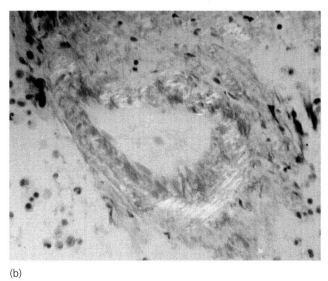
(b)

Fig. 11.1 Amyloidosis in bone marrow. (a) H&E. (b) Congo red under polarized light.

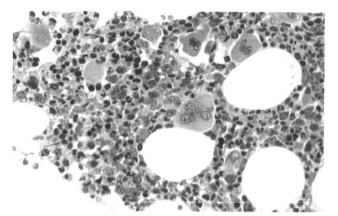

Fig. 11.2 Increased numbers of small megakaryocytes in chronic immune thrombocytopenic purpura (ITP). Giemsa.

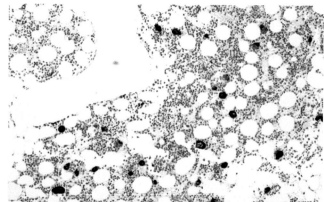

Fig. 11.3 Increased numbers of megakaryocytes in ITP are easier to detect by immunostaining (CD31 in this case).

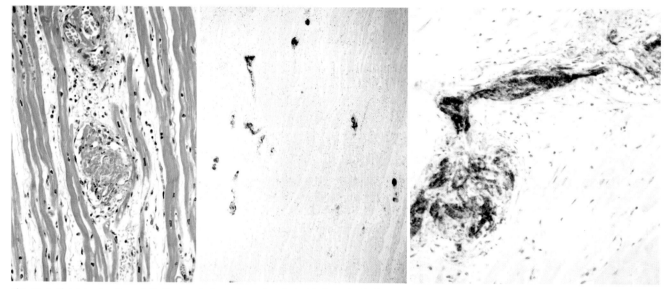

Fig. 11.4 Platelet microthrombi in the heart of a patient who died with thrombotic thrombocytopenic purpura (TTP).

It is generally easy to distinguish ITP from myelodysplasia and myeloproliferation by its lack of architectural and cytologic abnormality.

Assessing the number of megakaryocytes in a marrow trephine can be performed by formal counting and normal ranges are quoted (12–25 megakaryocytes per square millimeter[1,2]). In practice, a significant increase (i.e. more than twice the normal upper range) in megakaryocyte numbers can be confidently identified with a little experience of trephine histology or by immunostaining (Fig. 11.3). The latter always highlights more megakaryocytes than the former so one's normal range needs to be adjusted accordingly.

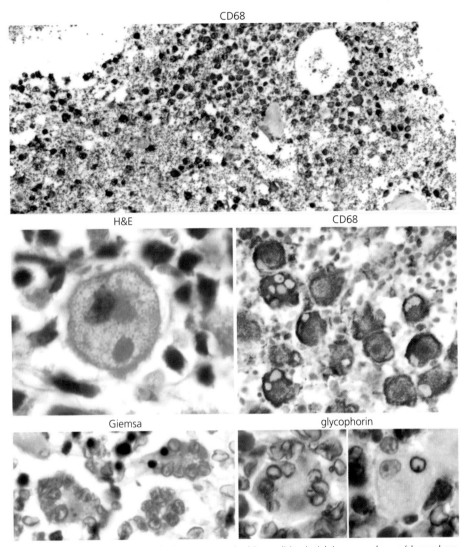

Fig. 11.5 Erythrophagocytosis: The bone marrow in this condition is rich in macrophages (shown here with CD68 immunostaining) most of which are full of red cells (demonstrated well with immunostaining for a red cell antigen such as glycophorin). They can also of course be seen with H&E and Giemsa staining.

Thrombotic thrombocytopenic purpura

Thrombotic thrombocytopenic purpura (TTP) has similarities to ITP above but is caused by a peripheral consumption of platelets caused by ill-defined underlying mechanisms often referred to as disseminated intravascular coagulation or vascular microangiopathy. The condition is associated with a range of factors very similar to those listed above for ITP. It is fortunately exceptionally rare as its acute form has an especially aggressive course. Patients, often young adults, develop multiple platelet-rich microthrombi in virtually all organs of the body and symptoms are largely related to the effects these have at those sites (Fig. 11.4). Bone marrow biopsy is not normally involved in management, which may account for variations in the description of the histology in these conditions from normal to hypercellular with megakaryocytic hyperplasia.

Erythrophagocytosis

Occasional examples of red cells phagocytosed by macrophages can be found in most marrows if one is prepared to spend the time looking. Erythrophagocytosis refers to those conditions (Table 11.1) where many if not the majority of the macrophages contain phagocytosed red cells, sometimes being stuffed with them (Fig. 11.5).

Table 11.1 Pathologic conditions often associated with erythrophagocytosis.

Viral infections (e.g. infectious mononucleosis)
Bacterial infections
Hemolytic anemia
AIDS
Familial erythrophagocytic lymphohistiocytosis
Malignancy (e.g. T cell lymphoma)
Post chemotherapy
Malignant histiocytosis
   (very rare and erythrophagocytosis is not prominent)

AIDS, acquired immunodeficiency syndrome.

Table 11.2 Causes of fibrosis in the bone marrow.

Common

Myeloproliferative disease
- Chronic primary myelofibrosis
- Acute myelofibrosis (acute megakaryoblastic leukemia)
- Polycythemia vera
- Essential thrombocythemia
- Chronic granulocytic leukemia

Hodgkin's disease (Hodgkin lymphoma)
Metastatic carcinoma

Less common

Acute leukemias
Treated acute leukemias
Systemic mastocytosis
Myelodysplasia
Non-Hodgkin lymphoma, e.g.
- Multiple myeloma
- Waldenström macroglobulinemia

Tuberculosis
Sarcoidosis
Scarring; following necrosis, previous biopsy, fracture, osteomyelitis
Paget disease
Renal osteodystrophy

Table 11.3 Causes of granulomas.

Infection	Sarcoidosis
Tuberculosis	*Malignant disease*
Atypical mycobacteria	Hodgkin disease
	(Hodgkin lymphoma)
Disseminated BCG	Multiple myeloma
Brucellosis	Non-Hodgkin lymphoma
Leprosy	Mycosis fungoides
Syphilis	ALL
Typhoid fever	MDS
Legionnaires disease	
Tularemia	*Drug hypersensitivity*
Q fever	Phenytoin
Rocky Mountain spotted fever	Procainamide
Leishmaniasis	Phenylbutazone &
	oxyphenylbutazone
Toxoplasmosis	Chlorpropamide
Histoplasmosis	Sulfasalazine
Cryptococcosis	Ibuprofen
Saccharomyces	Indomethacin
Blastomycosis	Allopurinol
Coccidioidomycosis	Interferon α-2b
Paracoccidioidomycosis	
Infectious mononucleosis	*Post-transplantation of*
	bone marrow
CMV	
Herpes zoster	*Associated with eosinophilic*
	interstitial nephritis
Hantaan virus	
Cat scratch fever	*Renal osteodystrophy*
Viral hepatitis	
	Reaction to foreign substances
	Anthracosis and silicosis
	Talc
	Berylliosis

ALL, acute lymphoblastic leukemia; BCG , Bacillus Calmette-Guerin ; CMV, cytomegalovirus; MDS, myelodysplastic syndrome.

Fibrosis

The causes of fibrosis in the bone marrow are numerous (Table 11.2). A semi-quantitative method of assessment is described in figure 2.9 (p. 8).

Granulomas

As with other tissues in the body, granulomas in the marrow can have a wide variety of appearances, ranging from occasional collections of a few epithelioid macrophages to fully formed granulomas consisting of tight clusters of epithelioid macrophages and multinucleated giant cells with a cuff of small lymphocytes. It is our experience that granulomas are easier to identify using H&E rather than Giemsa which tends to stain epithelioid macrophages poorly (Fig. 11.6). There are numerous causes (Table 11.3) for granuloma formation and the pathologist can often only provide a differential diagnosis relevant to the clinical details. In a percentage of cases no cause will ever be found.

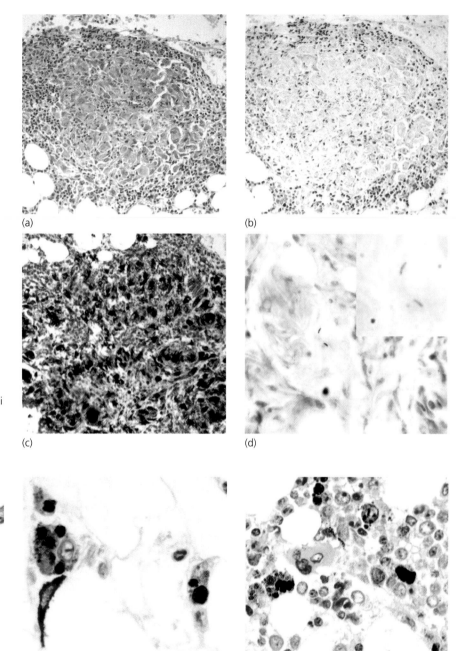

Fig. 11.6 Granuloma in bone marrow. (a) H&E. (b) Giemsa. (c) Immunostain for CD68 (macrophage marker) (d) Typical tubercle bacilli (at higher power in insert) seen in epithelioid macrophage: Ziehl-Neelsen stain.

(a)　　　　　(b)　　　　　(c)

Fig. 11.7 Iron in macrophages following blood transfusion. (a) H&E. (b,c) Giemsa.

Hemosiderin

Hemosiderin can be detected in both H&E and Giemsa stained sections. It takes the form of fine and coarse granules that appear brown on H&E and olive green on Giemsa stained sections (Fig. 11.7).

The granules are present within macrophages and may be associated with erythroid colonies. Decalcification of the biopsy may reduce the amount of iron so that assessment of iron content is best carried out on the aspirate smear. A semi-quantitative method of assessing iron content is shown in Table 11.4.

The most commonly encountered conditions that may affect iron stores are listed in Table 11.5.

Table 11.4 Semi-quantitative grading scheme for hemosiderin in tissue section. After Krause *et al.*[3]

Grade	Appearance
0	No iron seen
1	Granules in 1 out of 3 high powered fields
2	Granules in 1 out of 2 high powered fields
3	A few granules in every high powered field
4	> A few granules in every high powered field

Table 11.5 Conditions affecting iron stores.

Lack of iron brought about by:
Chronic disease
Inadequate diet
Chronic bleeding
Polycythemia vera

Excess iron brought about by:
Aplasia
Leukemia
Multiple transfusions (e.g. thalassemia)
MDS
Chronic disease with impaired iron handling and accumulation in macrophages

MDS, myelodysplastic syndrome.

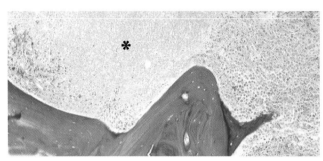

Fig. 11.8 Necrosis: transition from viable leukemia cells to total necrosis (*). Giemsa.

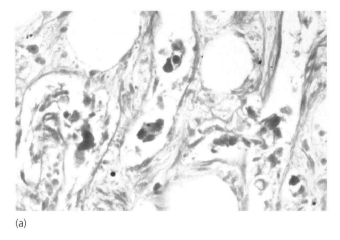

(a)

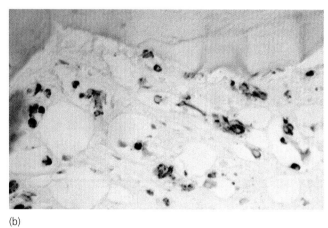

(b)

Fig. 11.9 Necrotic carcinoma cells in bone marrow can be clearly identified by immunostaining for cytokeratins. (a) H&E. (b) Immunostain for cytokeratins.

Necrosis

When examining a marrow trephine, it is important to make the distinction between:

1 Necrosis involving the bone and marrow, such as is seen in sickle cell disease, embolism, caisson disease (the "bends"), sepsis.

2 Necrosis predominantly affecting the marrow tissue, which is almost invariably associated with malignancy, such as acute leukemia, non-Hodgkin lymphoma, Hodgkin's disease (Hodgkin lymphoma) and metastatic carcinoma. If the tumor load in the marrow is high and there is massive necrosis then the bone may also become involved. Dead bone is identified by loss of the osteocyte population.

The necrotic cells show the features of necrosis seen in any tissue. The cells initially have darkly staining pyknotic nuclei that later disintegrate as karyorrhexis and karyolysis occurs. The cytoplasm is smudgy and eosinophilic. The overall impression is of ghost-like cells lacking any sharp well-defined features. Areas of fibrosis may be seen as healing occurs (Fig. 11.8).

Immunohistochemistry may be useful in identifying the nature of the dead cells (e.g. anti-cytokeratin antibodies have been shown to be useful in this respect). Care must be taken in interpretation of immunohistochemistry because of the increased tendency for antibodies to adhere in a non-specific way to necrotic tissue (Fig. 11.9).

Osteoporosis

Osteoporosis is a decreased amount of bone per unit volume. This results in a reduction in the amount of trabecular bone seen in a tissue section by a thinning of the trabeculae. Morphometry of bone will allow an accurate assessment of bone trabecular thickness but as a general rule a trabecula is at least the width of a fat cell. However, trabecular thickness varies individually and unless the condition is severe it is not that easy to identify osteoporosis in a routine trephine. A useful guide comes from a trephine where the bones are fragmented (because they are so weak) but the rest of the marrow is well preserved (indicating good technical preservation). Usually, in these cases the clinician has already identified the condition by its feel at biopsy (Fig. 11.10).

Osteoporotic change is most frequently seen in the elderly population especially in women. It is also seen in bones no longer stimulated by normal weight-bearing activities (e.g. patients who are immobilized).

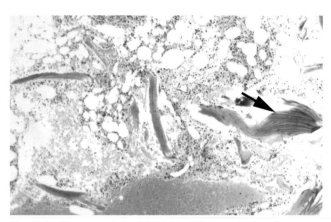

Fig. 11.10 Osteoporosis: typical thin easily fractured trabeculae. Note the osteoid seams are relatively normal (arrow). Giemsa.

Less common causes include endocrine disorders, long-term steroid administration and certain malignancies (e.g. multiple myeloma).

Renal osteodystrophy

Renal osteodystrophy or renal bone disease is caused by the metabolic changes associated with chronic renal failure such as hypocalcemia and secondary hyperparathyroidism. This is a complex bony abnormality which may include the changes of osteomalacia, osteitis fibrosa cystica, osteoporosis and osteosclerosis, either singly or in combinations.

Bone marrow biopsies from patients with chronic renal failure may show a number of histologic changes related to this constellation of conditions. There is usually evidence of increased destruction of bone and increased production. These structural changes are seen in association with abnormal cellular activity in the form of increased osteoblasts and osteoclasts. The bone trabeculae may have "tunnels" excavated within them by osteoclasts. These are essentially exaggerated forms of Howship lacunae. These newly created spaces, and eventually the intertrabecular spaces containing the marrow, may be filled with vascularized fibrous tissue. The osteoblasts lay down new bone which is of the woven variety and there is an increase in the amount of osteoid (not apparent in decalcified sections). In extreme cases the appearances of osteodystrophy may resemble Paget disease of the bone, although in the latter case the trabeculae are generally thicker and a mosaic pattern of cement lines is evident.

The marrow itself is unremarkable or shows erythroid hyperplasia and there may be increased hemosiderin from multiple blood transfusions for anemia (Fig. 11.11).

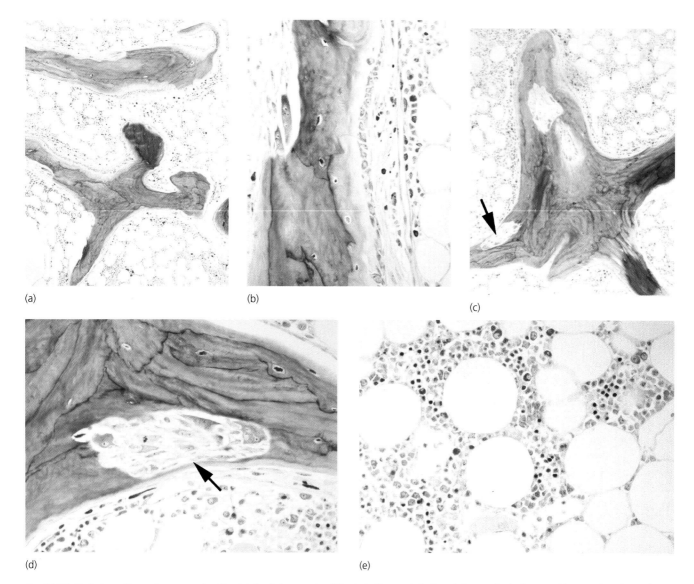

(a)   (b)   (c)

(d)   (e)

Fig. 11.11 Typical renal bone disease; see text for details of changes. (a–d) illustrate the constellation of changes in the bones with examples of tunneling (arrows) in c,d. (e) is a higher power of the marrow showing mild erythroid hyperplasia. Giemsa.

Paget disease

Paget disease is of unknown etiology and affects 3–4% of the population over the age of 45 years. Probably less than 5% of cases are symptomatic and may present as bone pain resulting from microfractures, deafness because of mechanical damage to the auditory nerve or, rarely, as cardiac failure. There is also an increased risk of developing osteogenic sarcoma.

The histologic features are:

1 Increased osteoclastic activity in the early stages with marked resorption of bone as evidenced by numerous Howship lacunae containing large multinucleated osteoclasts.

2 This is followed by bone hyperplasia undertaken by increased numbers of osteoblasts. The bone is laid down, originally as woven bone and then as lamellar bone. This results in thickened trabeculae with disjointed, multidirectional cement lines: the so-called mosaic pattern.

3 Within the marrow space there is an increase in the vascularity, which if extensive can act as an arteriovenous shunt resulting occasionally in high output cardiac failure (Fig. 11.12).

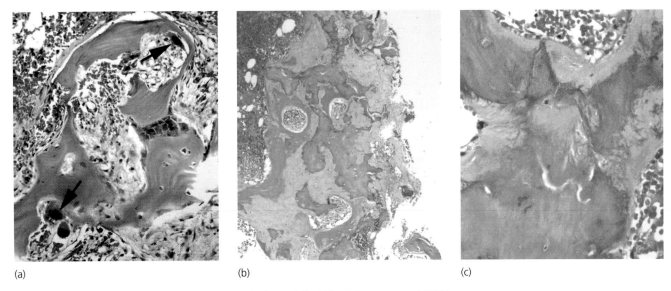

(a)   (b)   (c)

Fig. 11.12 Paget disease. (a) Increased osteoclastic activity (arrows). (b,c) Mosaic bone pattern. All H&E.

H&E

Giemsa

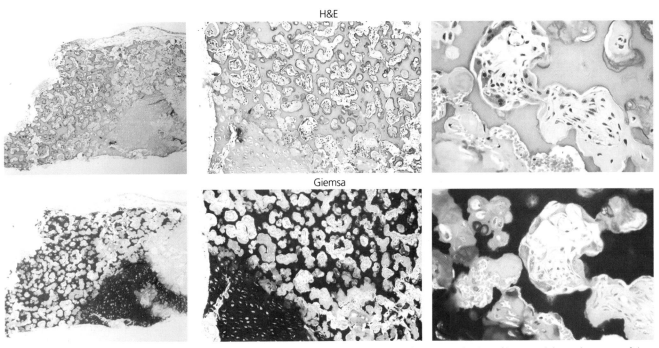

Fig. 11.13 Osteopetrosis shown at several magnifications with both H&E and Giemsa. Note the overproduction of bone and the replacement of the marrow spaces by fibrotic tissue. Osteoclasts are present but do not work properly.

Osteopetrosis

This is a genetic metabolic bone disease caused by defective bone resorption brought about by defective osteoclastic function. It is known from its radiologic features as "marble bone disease", a term well understood by any hematologist trying to extract a biopsy from these extremely hard bones (Fig. 11.13).

Clinical symptoms are caused by progressive replacement of the marrow spaces with bone and fibrosis leading to progressive pancytopenia with extramedullary hematopoiesis. The severity of the disease is variable with autosomal recessive forms often being lethal *in utero* while some autosomal dominant types have minimal symptoms. Some good therapeutic results have been reported from bone marrow transplantation.

Table 11.6 Causes of serous atrophy
(gelatinous transformation of the marrow).

AIDS
Cancer
Chronic renal disease
Irradiation
TB
Anorexia nervosa
Chemotherapy
Hypothyroidism
Malabsorption

AIDS, acquired immunodeficiency syndrome; TB, tuberculosis.

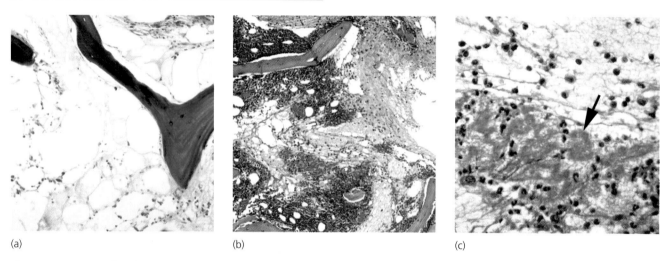

(a) (b) (c)

Fig. 11.14 Serous atrophy in bone marrow. (a) Giemsa. (b) H&E. (c) Amyloid-like aggregations (arrow). H&E.

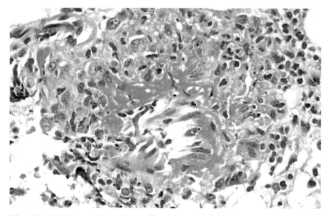

Fig. 11.15 Polyarteritis nodosa affecting arteriole in bone marrow. H&E.

Serous atrophy

This has also been termed gelatinous transformation and serous degeneration. It was originally described in patients with anorexia nervosa but may be seen in anyone with rapid marked loss in body weight (Table 11.6). Nowadays it is fre-

Table 11.7 Conditions in which foamy macrophages may be seen.

Sepsis (e.g. occasionally seen in ITU patients)
Fat necrosis (e.g. may be related to previous biopsy at that site)
Hyperlipidemia
Pseudo-Gaucher cells
Inherited disorders
• Gaucher disease
• Niemann–Pick disease
• Fabry disease
• Batten disease
Langerhans cell histiocytosis

AIDS, acquired immunodeficiency syndrome; TB, tuberculosis.

quently seen in patients with AIDS who have had severe weight loss. The changes are usually focal with the marrow fat cells being surrounded and gradually replaced by an extracellular homogeneous fibrillary pale material which is rich in hyaluronic acid. On H&E stained sections it has a smoky lilac color, sometimes with brighter red aggregations which should be distinguished from amyloid (Fig. 11.14).

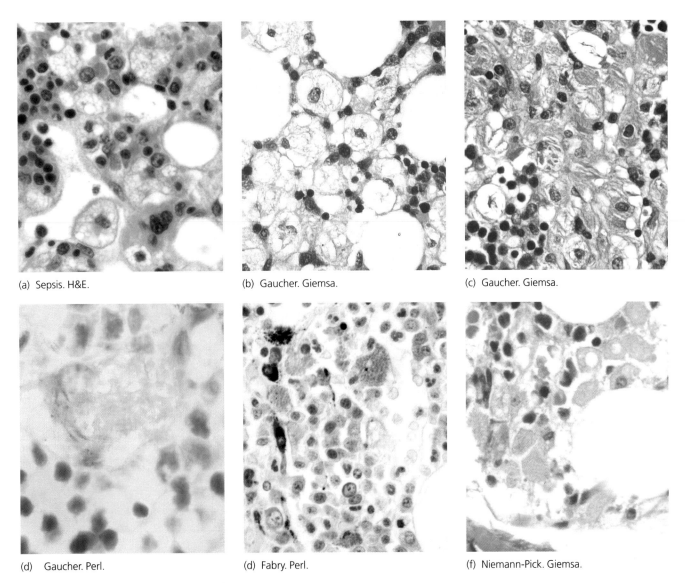

(a) Sepsis. H&E.

(b) Gaucher. Giemsa.

(c) Gaucher. Giemsa.

(d) Gaucher. Perl.

(d) Fabry. Perl.

(f) Niemann–Pick. Giemsa.

Fig. 11.16 Foamy macrophages in various conditions.

Vasculitis

The marrow has a rich blood supply and contains a range of blood vessel types, including small arteries, which are susceptible to the same diseases that affect blood vessels elsewhere in the body. It is not particularly well endowed with the medium to large vessels, which are more commonly affected by the major forms of vasculitis so the trephine rarely yields a positive diagnosis. Occasionally, it can be helpful or even diagnostic in conditions such as polyarteritis nodosa (Fig. 11.15).

Foamy macrophages

Foamy macrophages are seen in a number of very different conditions (Table 11.7). In severe sepsis the macrophages contain lipid vacuoles, presumably derived from erythrocyte membrane degradation. Hemosiderin may also be present (Fig. 11.16).

Inherited lipid storage disorders are characterized by the presence of foamy macrophages sometimes filling the marrow as in Gaucher disease or scattered focally as in Niemann–Pick or Fabry disease. In certain hematologic malignancies, particularly chronic myeloid leukemia, cells resembling Gaucher cells ("pseudo-Gaucher cells") have been described although in our experience they are not a prominent or common feature.

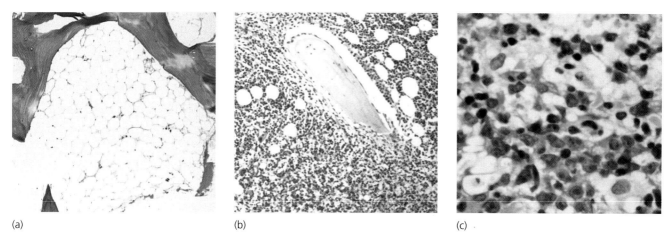

(a)　　　　　　　　　　　　　　(b)　　　　　　　　　　　　　　(c)

Fig. 11.17 (a) Aplasia resulting from exposure to solvent-based paint thinners. H&E. (b,c) Pseudolymphomatous hyperplasia from phenytoin. H&E.

The effects of drugs and chemicals

Drugs and chemicals have a variety of effects on the marrow which are beyond the scope of this text (and these authors!). In many cases the changes are non-specific (e.g. excessive intake of alcohol may produce an increase in the numbers of plasma cells and mast cells within the marrow). Others are more dramatic such as the striking aplasia that can be induced by solvent exposure or the pseudolymphomatous changes of phenytoin. Perhaps the most important point to make is to consider the drug history with any marrow changes inexplicable on other grounds (Fig. 11.17).

References

1 Ellis JT, Peterson P. The bone marrow in polycythemia vera. In: Sommers JC (ed). *Pathology Annual*, Vol. 14, Part 1. New York: Appleton-Century-Crofts, 1979, pp. 383–403.

2 Branehög I, Kutti J, Ridell B, *et al.* The relation of thrombokinetics to bone marrow megakaryocytes in idiopathic thrombocytopenic purpura. *Blood* 1975; **45**: 551–62.

3 Krause JR, Brubaker DO, Kaplan J. Comparison of stainable iron in aspirated and needle biopsy specimens of bone marrow. *Am J Clin Pathol* 1979; **72**: 68–70.

Chapter 12 Technical considerations

The debate over whether trephines should be embedded in paraffin wax or plastic resin will doubtless continue for some time. We have reviewed this in some detail in Chapter 1 and given our reasons for believing that paraffin embedding is more satisfactory for routine diagnosis. The following technical considerations mainly relate to marrow biopsies that have been embedded in paraffin wax.

Preparation of bone marrow biopsies

Whatever methods are used in preparing marrow biopsies, it is essential that:
- there be effective fixation of the tissue to ensure that good morphology is retained and that the bone is processed to enable sections of 2–4 μm to be cut;
- a range of special staining techniques (e.g. Giemsa, reticulin) remain applicable;
- tissue antigenicity is not adversely affected by procedures so that immunohistochemical techniques are applicable.

Both the bone marrow trephine biopsy and bone marrow aspirate (i.e. clot specimen) may be used to examine the state of the marrow. The following is the fixation and processing procedure used on the majority of the specimens in this book but any technique that gives good results as above is fine. Other fixatives such as Bouin or B5 give very good results as does ethylenediaminetetra-acetic acid (EDTA) as a decalcifying agent. Indeed, the latter may have some advantage over acids in preserving nucleic acid structures for molecular examination should this be required.

Fixation
Fixative

All specimens are fixed in 2% formol-acetic:
- Formaldehyde, 40% w/v   1 L
- Water   9 L
- Sodium chloride   87 g
- Glacial acetic acid   200 mL

Duration of fixation

Aspirates: fixation of aspirate specimens is complete after 24 hours. The particles are embedded in 1–2% agar and processed as tissue blocks.

Trephines: trephine specimens should be fixed for 48–72 hours and over this period the solution changed at least three times, more frequently if the trephine is large or there is a lot of bone. This is satisfactory for most specimens.

Occasionally, trephines are received containing a relatively large amount of solid bone or cartilage which proves an obstacle to satisfactory sectioning. In such cases, that part of the core can be separated from the remainder of the tissue because it is unlikely to contain cells of diagnostic significance.

If the core contains spicules of bone that remain heavily calcified, surface decalcification (with Perenyi fluid) after embedding may ease the situation although this must be done judiciously to prevent damage to tissue morphology or antigenicity.

Processing and embedding

Specimens are processed to paraffin wax on an automated processor using an overnight schedule (15–18 hours). They are then blocked out in paraffin wax before sectioning on a conventional microtome (Rotary, Sledge, Base sledge) at 2–4 μm using disposable blades (Feather).

Staining of bone marrow biopsies

A standard H&E stain is usually satisfactory. For Giemsa staining the authors use the following recipe. As in cookery, good results require fine ingredients but will reward skill and patience.

Giemsa stain

1 Dewax and rehydrate sections (2–4 μm).
2 Wash in distilled water.
3 Place slides in Giemsa working solution for 1 hour. Stock solution: Giemsa's stain, BDH/Gurr product 35014. Working solution: dilute stock solution 1 : 4 with distilled water.
4 Wash well in water.
5 Commence differentiation by agitation in freshly prepared acetic acid solution (i.e. 100 mL distilled water) to which 6–8 drops of glacial acetic acid has been added. Section will appear deep pink when this phase is complete.
6 Transfer directly to 95% IMS (industrial methylated spirit) and with gentle agitation, complete differentiation.
7 Halt differentiation by rinsing in isopropyl alcohol.
8 Clear in xylene.
9 Mount in DPX (mounting medium—BDH).

Immunohistochemistry

Pretreatment

About 10 years ago the introduction of heat treatment, microwaving and pressure cooking revolutionized our ability to detect antigens in routinely fixed sections. Our laboratory, like many others, made great efforts to establish which were the optimal conditions for each antibody, which we recorded in our table of useful antibodies in the first edition of this book. Since then there have been several other minor advances, most notably the introduction of several buffering solutions which one can either make up oneself or purchase. These can be used alone or in conjunction with any of the heat retrieval techniques. We have also discovered, as have most of our colleagues, that there is no one best method and that a certain element of trial and error may be needed. Our technique with any new antibody is to try it with and without microwaving or pressure cooking and then experiment from there. Frankly, the number of available options is beyond the scope of this book and would turn more into a cookery manual than a diagnostic album if we were not careful. Fortunately, there is a mass of commercial literature freely available and several excellent websites such as www.ihcworld.com. They all come up with results quickly with a search such as "antigen retrieval" on Google or other search engines. We believe it better to leave others to decide the best conditions for themselves but here leave in the sections detailing exactly how we microwave and pressure cook.

Microwaving

Tissue antigenicity can be enhanced by enzyme digestion and microwave heating or pressure cooking. It is therefore advisable to cut sections onto slides coated with an adhesive such as silane.

A suggested methodology for microwave retrieval of antigens that are not normally detectable in standard processed material is given below:
1 Dewax and rehydrate sections. If a technique incorporating a peroxidase label is used, block endogenous enzyme activity as usual.
2 Wash in distilled water.
3 Place slides in glass rack in a Pyrex dish and immerse in sufficient solution to cover slides:

    0.01 M sodium citrate, $Na_3C_6H_5O_7 2H_2O$ (2.94 g/L)
    0.01 M sodium bicarbonate, $NaHCO_3$ (0.84 g/L)
    0.01 M HCl/sodium citrate buffer, pH 6.0
    33 mL 0.01 M sodium citrate + 17 mL 0.01 M HCl
    Cover dish with microwave-proof clingfilm. Puncture to allow steam to escape.

4 Microwave for 5 minutes at full power. Check fluid level; top up as necessary. Microwave for a further 5 minutes at full power. Remove from oven and allow slides to stand for 10–15 minutes in the hot solution.
5 Wash in distilled water and then in buffer. Proceed with immunocytochemical technique.

Disadvantages and limitations

- Sections are easily detached during the microwaving procedure. Slides coated with silane or poly-L-lysine must be used.
- Denaturation of tissue may occur, resulting in unrecognizable morphology, if exposed for excessive periods or if tissue is fixed in solutions other than formalin.
- With some antibodies the treatment leads to staining distributions greater than that seen by other techniques, suggesting this may be artefactual.
- The method is not suitable for use with all antibodies. It appears that heating rather than the action of microwaves is the important feature, although heating in distilled water has little effect. Heating in a pressure cooker or an autoclave gives similar results.

Table 12.1 Suggested antibody types for identifying normal cells.

Normal cell types	Antibody
Megakaryocytes and precursors	CD61, CD31, factor VIII-related antigen
Erythroid cells	Glycophorin A or C
Granulocytes	Neutrophil elastase, myeloperoxidase or CD15
Monocytes	CD68 or CD163
Plasma cells	CD138, VS38 (p63 plasma cell antigen), κ & λ light chains
Lymphocytes	Leukocyte common antigen CD45
Vessels	CD31, CD34 or factor VIII-related antigen

Pressure treatment
(using a standard domestic pressure cooker)

1 Dissolve 5.88 g sodium citrate in 2 L of distilled water and correct pH to 6.0.

2 Pour the citrate buffer into the pressure cooker.

3 Place the lid loosely on the body of the pan and heat to a "rolling boil."

4 When a "rolling boil" occurs, place the slides into the boiling buffer.*

5 Seal the pan and ensure that the cook control is in the manual position.

6 The emergency pressure seal will soon rise, but it is necessary to wait another 5–8 minutes until the metal part of the Rise "N" Time indicator has risen (a clear indicator that the correct temperature has been reached.)

7 Fill sink with cold water.

8 Once the Rise "N" Time indicator has risen, time for 90 seconds.

9 Reduce pressure by immediately placing pan in sink and flushing the lid with cold tap water.

10 Once hissing stops and the emergency seal falls back, lid can be opened; fill pan to the brim with cold water before removing slide racks.

NB Boiling fluid at pressure can lead to severe burns if mishandled. If in difficulty, leave pan on hotplate, turn off heat and do not return to pan until pressure has subsided.

The value of immunostaining methods

Alkaline phosphatase methods are particularly suited to bone marrow specimens because of their high amount of endogenous peroxidase activity. With careful suppression, equally high quality results are readily obtainable with immunoperoxidase methods. Most immunostaining procedures can be adapted to trephines and laboratories should refer to their antibody suppliers for advice and technical support.

Remember that relatively few antibodies are absolutely specific for individual cell types. It is important for the pathologist to consult the specification sheet enclosed with these products or original papers before using new antibodies and it is always a good idea to perform stainings with a panel of antibodies to ensure that exceptions to general rules are observed. For example, a small number of malignant melanomas and anaplastic large cell lymphomas express cytokeratins. If appropriate confirmatory stains are not included, an incorrect diagnosis of carcinoma may be made.

Below we have attempted to cover those areas of diagnostic pathology where immunohistochemistry may be most usefully applied.

1 Assessment of cellularity
2 Dry tap
3 Focal disease
4 Classification of lymphoma and leukemia.

Assessment of cellularity

It is often useful to give clinicians accurate information on the cellular make-up of particular marrow samples (e.g. the ratio of residual marrow cells to malignant infiltrate and the assessment of a bone marrow prior to harvest for autologous transplantation). There are a number of antibodies that are very useful in labeling individual cell lines of the hematopoietic tissue (Table 12.1).

Dry tap

A dry tap means that on aspiration of the bone, no marrow cells are obtained so that a trephine needs to be taken if diagnostic material is required. Dry tap is generally explained by a fibrotic reaction in the marrow or an increase in cellularity sufficient to prevent aspiration (i.e. a "packed" marrow). Table 12.2 outlines the main causes of these and lists easily available antibody types which will assist in diagnosis.

* Four racks can be used at once in most pressure cookers.

Table 12.2 Causes and diagnoses of dry taps.

Cause of dry tap	Diagnosis	Antibody types
Fibrosis	Secondary carcinoma	Cytokeratin, epithelial membrane antigen
	Neuroblastoma	Neuroblastoma-associated antigen (NB84)
	Rhabdomyosarcoma	Desmin or myoglobin
	Hodgkin disease	CD15 or CD30
Hypercellular	Lymphoma	See section on Classification of lymphoma and leukemia
	Leukemia	See section on Classification of lymphoma and leukemia
	Reactive*	CD61 ? megakaryocytes
		Myeloperoxidase ? granulocytes
		Glycophorin A or C ? erythroid
		p63 antigen ? plasma cells

Table 12.3 Some causes of focal disease in bone marrows.

Non-Hodgkin lymphoma, especially follicular and CLL (see Table 12.4)
Hodgkin lymphoma (see Table 12.2)
Carcinoma (see Table 12.2)

CLL, chronic lymphocytic leukemia.

Focal disease

Foci of malignant disease often cause diagnostic problems either because they are not aspirated or not spread out into the smear. Some causes of focal disease in bone marrows are shown in Table 12.3. One special problem in this area is to distinguish reactive from malignant lymphoid nodules. There is no easy solution to this problem, especially if the nodules are small and composed mainly of well-differentiated small lymphocytes. Here the only test of value is to demonstrate light chain clonality, which cannot always be performed reliably regardless of the expertise of the individual laboratory.

Classification of lymphoma and leukemia

Lymphoma classification is a complex area and differs depending on the exact scheme used by different pathologists. Table 12.4 is an outline of the results that can be achieved by immunostaining which will be of assistance in establishing the general categories of lymphomas that are recognized by most lymphoma diagnosticians. For example, most schemes now accept that lymphomas should be divided into T or B cell types. For further details consult Chapter 8.

Antibodies for diagnostic use and the CD system

Throughout this text we have referred to antigens where possible by using their CD designation. CD stands for "cluster of differentiation" and represents an internationally agreed system for classifying antigens and their respective monoclonal antibodies. A CD group is a cluster of antibodies recognizing the same antigen. Where there is a series of related genes giving rise to antigenic variants the CD groups have been subdivided (e.g. CD1 a, b, c or CD11 a and b). These groupings are defined at International Workshops on Human Leucocyte Differentiation Antigens. The first of these was held in Paris in 1982, when 15 CD groups were defined. There have to date been eight workshops and the number of clusters has increased to 247. Although this seems a large number it is nothing compared with the thousands of antibodies, each with their own "laboratory" names, which have been allocated to the clusters. Thus, referring to the CD number of an antibody rather than the "pet" name used by the laboratory that produced it (e.g. CD30 rather than Ber H2) allows greater clarity and understanding between users of immunohistochemistry. There are many important antigens with perfectly good names recognized by reliable antibodies that do not have CD numbers. One should not fall into the trap of thinking these are in some way inferior. Table 12.5 is a summary of the antigens and antibodies that we have found helpful in bone marrow diagnosis. Interested parties can discover more about the CD system from the relevant workshop reports or about any of these antibodies from a number of antibody companies which have information fact sheets available (e.g. R&D Systems, DAKO a/s or visionbiosystems). All have websites and in addition there are many antibody search and review sites also available on the web.

Table 12.4 Immunocytochemical aids in lymphoma and leukemia diagnosis.

	Antibody types
Lymphoma	
Lymphoid origin	Leukocyte common antigen positive (except many anaplastic large cell lymphomas which are negative)
High or low grade	Ki-67 antigen (monoclonal and polyclonal)
B cells	CD20, CD79a, PAX5
T cells	CD3
ALC	CD30 and ALK
Myeloma	Plasma cell antigen (p63, CD38 or CD138), κ and λ light chains
Leukemia	
cALL	CD79a, CD10, TdT
T ALL	CD3, TdT
AML	Myeloperoxidase, CD117 (c-kit), CD68/CD163, CD34
CML	Abnormal cells of multiple lineage
Other rare leukemias	Identify by cell of origin (see section on Focal disease)

ALC, anaplastic large cell lymphoma; AML, acute myeloid leukemia; cALL, common acute lymphoblastic leukemia; CML, chronic myeloid leukemia; T ALL, T cell acute lymphoblastic leukemia.

Table 12.5 Antigens identifiable in routine trephine sections by commercially available antibodies.

Antigen	Suggested clone	Antigen	Suggested clone
Hematopoietic markers		Epithelial membrane antigen	E29
CD2	271	Factor VIII-related antigen	F8/86
CD3	Polyclonal	Hairy cell leukemia	DBA 44, TRAP(ZY-9C5)
CD4	NCL-CD4-1F6	κ/λ light chains	Polyclonal
CD5	4c7	Ki-67 antigen	Mib-1
CD7	272	Cyclin D1	Rabbit monoclonal SP4
CD8	C8/144B	Bcl2	124
CD10	270	Bcl6	Pg-b6p
CD15	C3D-1	Mast cell tryptase	AA1
CD20	L26	Myoglobin	Polyclonal
CD23	MHM6	Myeloperoxidase	Polyclonal
CD30	Ber-H2	Neutrophil elastase	NP57
CD31	JC70A	Plasma cell p63	VS38
CD34	QBend 10	TdT	339
CD45	2B11 and PD7/26	TIA-1	TIA-1<
CD56	1b6		
CD61	Y2/51		
CD68	KP1 or PGM1	*Non-hematopoietic markers*	
CD79a	JCB117	Desmin	D33
CD99 (mic2)	12e7	Neuroblastoma	NB84
CD117 (cKit)	Polyclonal	Cytokeratin (pan)	MNF116+LP34
CD138	MI 15	Cytokeratin 7	Ov-tl 12/30
CD163	10D6	Cytokeratin 20	Ks20.8
CD235 (Glycophorin A)	JC159/JC170	Prostate-specific antigen	Er-pr8
CD236 (Glycophorin C)	Ret40f	Estrogen receptor	ID5
CD246 (ALK)	ALK-1	Progesteron receptor	PgR636

Index